ISSUES AND MANAG

JOINT
HYPERMOBILITY

**A Guide for the Ehlers-Danlos Syndrome Hypermobility Type
and the Hypermobility Syndrome**

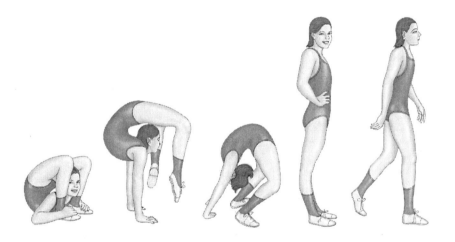

BRAD T. TINKLE, MD, PHD

Issues and Management of Joint Hypermobility: A Guide for the Ehlers-Danlos Syndrome Hypermobility Type and the Hypermobility Syndrome

International Standard Book Number: 978-0-9818360-0-3

Library of Congress Catalog Card Number: 2008933106

Printed in the United States of America

First Printing August 2008

Design and production by LOI International, a brand of Lauren Originals, Inc.

Published and distributed by Left Paw Press. For individual, educational, corporate, or retail sales accounts, email: customerservice@leftpawpress.com. For information address Left Paw Press, PO BOX 133, Greens Fork, IN 47345. Left Paw Press can be found on the web at www.leftpawpress.com.

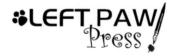

Contents

Foreword

A comprehensive guide for the treatment of generalized joint hypermobility (i.e. double-jointed) as part of one of the systemic connective tissue diseases (affecting many aspects of the whole body) such as one of the Ehlers-Danlos syndromes or the hypermobility syndrome is difficult to find. Many of those affected wait years and see multiple healthcare providers before some of the symptoms are recognized as features of an overall disorder. Several look well at the time- some may have joint hypermobility at present while others only a history of hypermobility as a youth. Countless others are diagnosed with secondary disorders such as fibromyalgia, chronic pain, and/ or depression without recognizing the underlying features of generalized joint hypermobility.

Healthcare providers are often poorly educated on the concerns of generalized joint hypermobility and other features that may complicate it. This leaves many patients frustrated, even after receiving a diagnosis, because features are not recognized as part of an overall syndrome. The information contained within this guide is from expert opinion and a compilation of the relevant medical literature. It is not meant to substitute as the plan for any individual patient as each person has unique needs. The information herein is meant for the general public including those affected, their family and friends as well as healthcare providers as initial "talking points" in developing the individual treatment plan. As we are continuing to learn more about EDS and the hypermobility syndrome, we expect that this information will continue to be refined and continue to evolve.

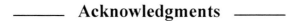

Acknowledgments

Many patients have struggled through the healthcare system and have learned what has worked for them and, equally as important, what has not. In hearing their stories and frustration, it is compelling to apply knowledge, experience, and an open mind to address their individual needs. Many researchers and clinicians have provided keen and very valuable insights into many aspects of these disorders, providing us the tools necessary to start addressing the needs of those affected. This is the foundation on which we will build.

Many others provided valuable time, experience, and compassion in the care of those affected. I want to thank most especially Ms. Carrie Atzinger as the backbone of the program at Cincinnati Children's Hospital Medical Center who serves as the program coordinator and a constant resource and inspiration. Similarly, prior program coordinators including Erin Miller and Leah Hoechstetter have lent their passion and hard work in the building of this program. Drs. Rick Wenstrup and Dick Meyer have been the cornerstones of this clinic and my inspiration. I also want to thank the many others who contribute to the evolving ideas in the care of such individuals. To name a few, I want to thank Paula Melson, Shannon Darnell, Opal Riddle, Dr. Victoria Surdulescu, Dr. Atiq Durrani, Dr. Sarah Lopper, Dr. Scott Pentiuk, Dr. Hammam Akbik, Dr. Patrick Agnew, Dr. Joseph Ernest III, and Dr. Nazli McDonnell.

I must also thank my wife for the inspiration and encouragement to put these thoughts to paper, completing a life goal of publishing a book of my own and fulfilling a need to promote patient and health professional education about EDS and the hypermobility syndrome.

1
——— Joint Laxity ———

Joint hypermobility or laxity refers to the increased movement (i.e., range of motion) of a particular joint, which is also commonly called "double-jointed." Many individuals have joint laxity at one or a few joints. This can be an inherited feature (family trait) but also can be due to training. As an example, musicians often have joint laxity of their fingers and gymnasts often have excessive laxity of several joints due to conditioning [O'Loughlin et al., 2008]. Generalized joint laxity refers to multiple joints, both small and large, that have hypermobility.

Generalized joint hypermobility is often determined using a particular scoring system based on physical examination. One of the most well known, widely-used, and rapid assessments is the Beighton criteria [Beighton et al., 1973]. The Beighton criteria evaluates excessive joint mobility in the small joints including the thumb and fifth finger (pinky), large joints such as the knees and elbows, as well as the spine [Figure 1.1]. Each joint can score one point, and therefore a total score of 9 points is possible. Because some people have joint laxity just isolated to small joints or large joints or their spine, generalized joint laxity is a score of 5 or greater which requires at least two types of joints to be involved.

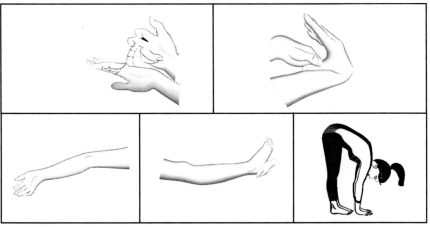

Figure 1.1. The maneuvers in the Beighton examination.

The Beighton exam consists of apposing the thumb to the forearm on each side [Figure 1.1]. If the thumb can touch the forearm, a score of 1 can be counted for each of the left and/or right side. Occasionally, patients can score positively on one side but not the other. This is most often due to the muscle bulk and use of that particular arm, usually based on the handedness (right or left) of the person [Pountain, 1992; Verhoeven et al., 1999]. The second criterion looks at the flexion of the fifth finger. If the fifth finger can be pulled backward <90°, it is considered a positive test. One point is given for each of left and/or right fifth finger. The assessment of the large joints includes hyperextension of the elbow with a fully outstretched arm. The elbow, when hyperextended, points upward, above the plane of the arm. If the angle created is >10° of hyperextension, this is considered a positive score. Females are more likely to have elbow hyperextension than males due to differences in the bone and muscle structure of the arm. Hyperextension of the knees is similar. Upon standing, if the knees can be forced backwards so that they extend beyond the line of the hip to the ankle >10° of hyperextension, this is also considered positive. It is difficult sometimes for the person to do this willingly. I have found, however, that if you ask patients to put their feet together when standing and to bend over, one can usually see the knees going backwards involuntarily (without thinking). For the final evaluation, the person stands flat footed, knees straight, and bends forward at the hips. If the person can touch the palms of their hands flat to the floor, it is considered positive. However, forward flexion of the spine may be restricted by pain in the back of the legs and lower back [Simmonds and Keer, 2008]. An overall score of 5 or greater indicates generalized joint hypermobility.

Unfortunately, joint hypermobility and therefore the Beighton score, is susceptible to many different problems. There are known changes in joint mobility with age such that younger children tend to be the most hypermobile. However, as we get older, our joints become stiffer. Therefore, the assessment of an adult is somewhat different than the assessment of a child. Even during childhood, joint laxity may be different (worse or better) during periods of growth as the ligaments are stretched before the muscles adapt [Bird, 2007]. Although joint laxity decreases with age, the pain that may be associated with it often progresses over time [Pountain, 1992; Ainsworth and Aulicino, 1993]. Loss of motion at any joint may occur due to pain-related disuse or to muscular imbalance. However, the Beighton scoring system does not account for many of these variables.

There is also a difference between the sexes. Women tend to be more flexible than men [Rowe et al., 1999; Gannon and Bird, 1999]. Up to 5% of healthy women have symptomatic joint hypermobility compared to only 0.6% of men [Engelbert et al., 2004]. This difference is likely due to several factors including: muscle build, skeletal features, activity-related differences between males and females, as well as hormonal influences. Joint laxity may increase in many women just prior to their period due to hormonal levels [Bird, 2007; Simmonds and Keer, 2008]. Similarly, joint laxity will also increase during pregnancy [Calguneri et al., 1982; Marnach et al., 2003].

Other variables also affect joint hypermobility. There can be differences between race and ethnicity. It has been found that Asians and African Americans are typically more hypermobile than Caucasians [Pountain, 1992; Verhoeven et al., 1999; Grahame and Hakim, 2008]. Lastly, joint hypermobility can be an acquired trait or maintained by activities that continue to stretch that joint such as in participating in dance, gymnastics, and the like.

Because the Beighton score is applied evenly yet there are many variables that potentially affect the scoring system, a healthcare provider experienced with joint hypermobility should use his/her best judgment. An adaptation of this scoring system, the Brighton criteria takes into account age-related joint stiffness [Table 1.1]. Therefore, a lower Beighton score is consistent with generalized joint hypermobility as long as a history of joint hypermobility is obtained upon questioning. Furthermore, the Brighton criteria takes into account symptoms related to joint hypermobility including chronic pain, dislocations (joint slipping in and out), and subluxations (excessive movement of the bone out of the joint).

Although the Beighton criteria can be used to diagnose generalized joint hypermobility, it does not distinguish between the different conditions that are associated with generalized joint hypermobility. Isolated and generalized joint laxity can be associated with other non-musculoskeletal features including such genetic syndromes as Ehlers-Danlos syndrome, Marfan syndrome, Stickler syndrome, Larsen syndrome, and osteogenesis imperfecta [Bird, 2007].

11

Table 1.1- Brighton revised diagnostic criteria for the hypermobility syndrome*

Major criteria
1. A Beighton score of 4/9 or greater (either currently or by history)
2. Pain for longer than 3 months in 4 or more joints

Minor criteria
1. A Beighton score of 1-3/9 if 50 years of age or older
2. Pain in 1-3 joints for 3 months (including the back), or spondylosis and/or spondylolisthesis
3. Dislocation/subluxation of more than 1 joint or in a single joint on more than one occasion
4. Soft tissue rheumatism at 3 sites including epicondylitis, tenosynovitis, and bursitis
5. Marfanoid habitus: tall, slim, span:height ratio >1.03, upper:lower segment ratio <0.89 (adult), and arachnodactyly
6. Abnormal skin: striae, hyperextensibility, thin skin, papyraceous scarring
7. Eye signs: drooping eyelids or near-sighted or down-slanting eyes
8. Varicose veins or hernia or uterine/rectal prolapse

Excluded in the presence of:
1. Marfan syndrome
2. Ehlers-Danlos syndrome other than the hypermobility type
The hypermobility syndrome is diagnosed in the presence of two major criteria **or** one major and two minor **or** four minor criteria or two minor criteria with an independently diagnosed first-degree relative.

*Adapted from Grahame et al., 2000

Link

Joint hypermobility, from the Arthritis Research Campaign
http://www.arc.org.uk/arthinfo/patpubs/6019/6019.asp

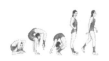

2
——— Ehlers- Danlos Syndromes ———

Ehlers-Danlos syndromes (EDS) are a group of inherited connective tissue diseases. There are 6 major subtypes [Table 2.1; Beighton et al., 1998].

Table 2.1 Types of Ehlers-Danlos Syndrome*			
Type	Formerly	Genetic defect	Clinical description
Classical	EDS I (gravis) EDS II (mitis)	Type V collagen in the majority of cases [Malfait et al., 2005]	Skin hyperextensibility; Widened atrophic scars; Hypermobile joint
Hypermobility	EDS III (hypermobile)	Largely unknown; Tenascin-X deficiency (rare)	Hyperextensible skin and/ or smooth and velvety skin; Joint hypermobility
Vascular	EDS IV (arterial-ecchymotic)	Type III collagen	Thin, translucent skin; Marked bruising; Rupture of arteries, uterus, or bowel; Characteristic facial appearance; Small joint laxity
Kyphoscoliotic	EDS VI (ocular-scoliotic)	Lysyl hydroxylase deficiency	Congenital scoliosis; Ocular fragility; Joint hypermobility; Hypotonia at birth
Arthrochalasia	EDS VII A/B (arthrochalasia multiplex congenita)	Type I collagen mutations affecting the N-proteinase cleavage site	Severe joint hypermobility; Stretchy skin; Increased risk of fractures
Dermatosparaxis	EDS VII C (human dermatosparaxis)	Deficiency of the procollagen N-proteinase	Joint hypermobility; Fragile sagging skin
*modified from Beighton et al., 1998			

Connective tissue provides structure to many organs as well as specific body parts. It has a major role in supporting muscles and bone. In general, EDS is characterized by a defect in connective tissue and these disorders commonly have joint hypermobility (i.e. "double-jointed") and unusual skin features.

Classic EDS has generalized joint hypermobility affecting small and large joints as well as skin that stretches farther than normal but instantly returns to its shape when released. However, the skin is fragile, wounds easily, heals poorly, and may leave abnormal scarring. At least half of the known cases are due to defects in type V collagen, whereas the genetic cause of the remaining cases are not known.

Hypermobile EDS (EDS-HM) is also an inherited disorder, but the genetic defect is largely unknown for this group. Patients will display generalized joint laxity, as well as soft, slightly distensible (i.e. stretchy) skin that may have some delayed healing but does not typically leave unusual scarring. It is often difficult to distinguish the mild classic form of EDS from the hypermobile form. Both the classic and the hypermobile forms of EDS have substantial joint instability which can result in frequent joint dislocations and/or subluxations (excessive movement of the bone out of the joint) resulting in pain as well as chronic joint damage. Many affected individuals experience significant joint pain often described as arthritic in nature, starting in their teens or early 20s. Those more severely affected may have had multiple dislocations and become physically limited. Although joint hypermobility is the common feature for classic and hypermobile EDS, as connective tissue affects multiple organs and tissue, there are a number of other additional features that will be discussed in detail elsewhere.

The **hypermobility syndrome** was initially described by Kirk et al. [1967] as excessive joint laxity that resulted in acute or chronic joint complaints but did not have features outside the musculoskeletal system and was not an inflammatory condition such rheumatoid arthritis or osteoarthritis. Over the following years, such patients were increasingly recognized as having other non-musculoskeletal concerns [Table 2.2]. Once called the benign joint hypermobility syndrome, it was soon recognized that the pain and other features constituted a significant medical disorder and has since been referred to as the hypermobility syndrome. It has been suggested that the hypermobility syndrome was a milder form of a connective tissue disease that should be distinguished from the Ehlers-Danlos syndromes. However, the distinction between the hypermobility syndrome and the hypermobile type of EDS cannot be readily made and many argue that they are one and the same [Bird, 2007; Levy, 2007; Grahame and Hakim, 2008]. I too, agree with this concept and will refer to both conditions as a single entity (EDS-HM).

Vascular EDS is due to defects in type III collagen. Patients with vascular EDS often have very thin skin that gives them a more aged appearance. They often have small joint laxity affecting the hands and feet but less frequently have large joint complications. Type III collagen provides a structural supporting role to a number of "hollow" organs including the stomach, intestines, bladder, and uterus in addition to blood vessels. The abnormal connective tissue results in weakened walls of organs or blood vessels, allowing the rupture of these walls. These events may be life-threatening in nature and often require very specific surgical management.

The **kyphoscoliotic type** of EDS is often seen as severe generalized joint hypermobility but such affected persons most often have a congenital (at birth) kyphoscoliosis (spinal deformity). Of equally great concern, the wall or globe of the eye is often thinned and weakened which can lead to rupture of the eye with little or no trauma.

see chart on next page...

Table 2.2- Brighton revised diagnostic criteria for the hypermobility syndrome*

Major criteria
1. A Beighton score of 4/9 or greater (either currently or by history)
2. Pain for longer than 3 months in 4 or more joints

Minor criteria1.
A Beighton score of 1-3/9 if 50 years of age or older
2. Pain in 1-3 joints for 3 months (including the back), or spondylosis and/or spondylolisthesis
3. Dislocation/subluxation of more than 1 joint or in a single joint on more than one occasion
4. Soft tissue rheumatism at 3 sites including epicondylitis, tenosynovitis, and bursitis
5. Marfanoid habitus: tall, slim, span:height ratio >1.03, upper:lower segment ratio <0.89 (adult), and arachnodactyly
6. Abnormal skin: striae, hyperextensibility, thin skin, papyraceous scarring
7. Eye signs: drooping eyelids or near-sighted or down-slanting eyes
8. Varicose veins or hernia or uterine/rectal prolapse

Excluded in the presence of:
1. Marfan syndrome
2. Ehlers-Danlos syndrome other than the hypermobility type

The hypermobility syndrome is diagnosed in the presence of two major criteria **or** one major and two minor **or** four minor criteria or two minor criteria with an independently diagnosed first-degree relative.

*Adapted from Grahame et al., 2000

The **arthrochalasia type** is often seen with dislocated hips and/or clubfeet (a foot deformity) at birth, severe generalized joint laxity, and skin findings typical of classic EDS. These patients may also have features of bone fragility (bones break easily) not seen in the other forms of EDS.

The **dermatosparaxis** form has more significant skin involvement with skin that is easily torn and sags but does not stretch back when pulled. Patients often have generalized joint hypermobility but this is somewhat mild in comparison.

Prior literature has described many other forms of EDS. These have been revised in the 1998 Villefranche Nosology to six major subtypes [Beighton et al., 1998]. Additional types may exist and are often classified as untypable EDS.

Diagnosis of EDS. The diagnosis of all types of EDS is most often clinical, based on physical features, most especially skin findings and joint hypermobility, as well as the medical and/or the family history of the person in question. Clinical diagnosis is often very reliable, if diagnosed by someone experienced in EDS. Family history of similar features is often helpful in delineating between the different types of EDS. Biochemical and/ or genetic testing is available for selected types, but should be used when the suspicion is based on clinical grounds. Often these manifestations are poorly recognized by healthcare providers not familiar with EDS [Adib et al., 2005]. Patients with EDS typically spend years before achieving the correct diagnosis and have seen multiple care providers before seeing someone familiar with EDS. Management is often symptomatic or preventative as there is no cure.

Links

Ehlers-Danlos syndrome, from Genetics Home Reference,
http://ghr.nlm.nih.gov/condition=ehlersdanlossyndrome/

Hypermobility, from Wikipedia,
http://en.wikipedia.org/wiki/Hypermobility

The Hypermobility Syndrome Association,
http://www.hypermobility.org/

Joint Hypermobility: An Information Booklet, from the Arthritis Research Campaign,
http://www.arc.org.uk/arthinfo/patpubs/6019/6019.asp

Marfan's Hypermobility Syndrome, Who Named It?
http://www.whonamedit.com/synd.cfm/954.html

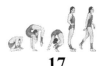

3
———— The Genetics of EDS-HM ————

EDS-HM is an inherited disorder of connective tissue, which is the tissue that provides structure to many organs as well as specific body parts. It follows an autosomal dominant pattern of inheritance. This means that an affected individual has a 50% chance of passing on this genetic trait to each of their children. In the conception of a baby, the mother and father contribute an equal amount of genetic material (genes). Therefore, each new baby is made up of genes given from the father and mother on an essentially equal basis. Autosomal refers to a number of genetic pairings that result without regard to the person's sex (gender). In such cases, for any given trait, the mother and the father contribute genetic traits equally. However, in dominant cases, one gene, either from the mother or the father, exerts a stronger influence over the genetic trait than the other and thus, will cause disease.

As each affected individual has a similar dominant and normal trait for the connective tissue disease, upon conceiving a child, this individual may pass on either the affected (dominant) or normal copy. Therefore, each individual has a 50% chance (1 out of 2) of passing on the genetic trait to future offspring. This is an independent risk meaning that if the individual already has one affected child, the next child still has a 50% chance of also being affected. However, unlike most genetic disorders, it is often very difficult to diagnose any newborn as to whether or not they have a connective tissue disease. In EDS-HM, there is no reliable test that can be performed either on a clinical basis (i.e. physical examination) or testing including genetic testing. As most infants, toddlers, and young children have joint laxity, it is often difficult to tell before the age of about six years, which child has excessive joint laxity in comparison to other children of their same age.

Males and females equally are at risk for having EDS-HM. However, males may have fewer symptoms such as pain or even joint laxity in comparison to a female sibling (sister). This is due in large part to the overall muscular build of a male versus female, the different types of activities that males often do versus females which require more strength versus more coordination, and subsequently, in the pre-teen years, due to female hormonal differences. It may be very difficult in some adults to determine whether they have had hypermobility as a child depending on their degree of joint hyperlaxity and symptoms. It is not unusual for a child to present with concerns of joint hypermobility, and upon either evaluation or detailed family history, one of the parents is also found to be hypermobile who may be essentially symptom-free or may have attributed their chronic joint pain to other conditions such as sports-related injuries and/or work-related activities.

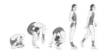

4
—— Pain ——

"Without pain medication, the pain is intolerable. It (pain medication) is the only thing that makes it possible to do physical therapy and do small tasks and socialize with family."

"In order to keep the pain level tolerable, I have to NOT do activities!"

Of 125 patients with joint pain and generalized joint hypermobility referred to a rheumatology clinic, Adib et al. (2005) found that only 10% of the referring physicians recognized that the hypermobility was the likely cause of the pain.

Pain is most often the initial complaint of someone with joint hypermobility [Adib et al., 2005] and is usually the most severe [Berglund and Nordstrom, 2001]. The pain may be intermittent or activity-related. Pain often progresses over time [Sacheti et al., 1997] despite decreasing joint mobility with age [Ainsworth and Aulicino, 1993]. Many adults live with constant pain that affect all aspects of their lives [Sacheti et al., 1997; Berglund et al., 2000].

Growing pains. Children with excessive joint laxity often complain of "growing pains." These are dull or throbbing aches typically around the knees or just above the knees that occur towards the end of the day and can lead to poor sleep. This may be due to stretching of the muscles during growth spurts. In addition, excessive joint laxity causes unusual wear in the joints and strains the muscles and ligaments supporting the joint and therefore, prolonged use (overuse) may cause pain. This will build up throughout the day and cause the typical intense and dull ache that children experience. It more often affects both sides but may show a preference of one side versus the other. Assessment by a doctor may be necessary but joint laxity-related pain is often overlooked and attributed to nonspecific growing pains in children.

Such pains related to hypermobility in small children should be treated differently. It is helpful to monitor the activities that help bring on the child's pain, such that longer periods of activity may be better to be interrupted, providing more rest, or the pace (speed) of the activity controlled more appropriately. If activities are known to cause pain, then giving ibuprofen (e.g. Advil® or Motrin®) prior to these activities will help with some of the pain later. Acetaminophen (e.g. Tylenol®) can be used in addition to the ibuprofen, specifically for pain after the activity. An often prescribed routine is: 1) appropriate dosing of ibuprofen prior to a day's activities such as extracurricular sports or days of prolonged physical activity including vacation days; 2) modification of activities where appropriate including the appropriate rest; and 3) acetaminophen when or if the pain persists following the activities.

It is encouraged that the child experiencing this pain on a recurring basis gets the appropriate rest between activities (for example, rest after practice). If adequate pain control cannot be achieved, then further interventions are required which may include significant restrictions/modification of activities, bracing, or increasing the pain medication. Additionally, physical therapy can be used to increase exercise tolerance and more appropriate use of joints during these activities. If the pain becomes daily, then a serious look at whether or not to continue these activities is necessary. Many children participate in sports and have significant pain associated with such activities. It may not be in the child's best interest to fully withdraw from activities, but if possible, modification of the activities is warranted. Chronic daily pain is best treated with chronic daily pain management that may include daily use of ibuprofen or appropriate pain medications. Chronic use of nonsteroidal anti-inflammatories (NSAIDs), such as ibuprofen, may cause stomach upset, heartburn, and nausea. Gastrointestinal (abdominal) complaints for patients with EDS are common and daily use of NSAIDs may worsen symptoms requiring additional use of "stomach" protective medications.

Adolescence. Pain often returns in the teen years associated with activities, typically involving the knees, hips, shoulders, and elbows. Frequent subluxations or dislocations may occur more often due to increased strength, which can cause significant pain. Often patients complain of daily pain, worse with activities and worsening throughout the day. Rest tends to help but as this continues, many wake up with dull aches the next morning as well (activity-related or pain "hangover"). Therapy is similar to that previously described for children including physical therapy with joint stabilization, postural training, bracing or orthotics as needed, as well as pain medication.

Often at this age, pain becomes chronic necessitating daily use of an anti-inflammatory medication (NSAIDs).

Location of pain. As multiple joints are involved, each has a predisposition to injury and pain. The painful sites are most often related to the activities of the person. A person with a "desk job" may complain more of hand and neck pain whereas those constantly on their feet complain of the weight-bearing joints such as the ankles, knees, and hips. The distribution and incidence of pain related to a body site among those affected with EDS-HM is reported in Table 4.1.

Pain medications: the tiered approach. NSAIDs are usually the first line of medication therapy as they help prevent further joint inflammation, damage, and pain. Since they do not directly affect pain, often other medications are needed for moderate to severe pain [Hunt et al., 2007]. A combination of ibuprofen and acetaminophen can be used for mild to moderate pain. A structured plan (a.k.a. a tiered approach) is used for different levels of pain. Often a chronic daily use of NSAIDs will be the first approach. Non-narcotics for mild to moderate breakthrough pain may include additional use of acetaminophen and possibly tramadol (Ultram®), which is a non-narcotic pain reliever [Altman, 2004; Brown and Stinson, 2004]. Many patients with chronic pain with mild to moderate flares may also benefit by regular use of medications used to treat neurologic pain including anti-seizure medications as well as antidepressants which often have additional benefits such as aiding sleep and mood. For moderate to severe pain, often combination products are used including acetaminophen and an opioid (a type of narcotic) [Raffa et al., 2003]. These must be used with caution when taken in addition to acetaminophen alone which can lead to overdose, liver damage, and death.

Table 4.1 - Bodily distribution of pain in EDS-HM					
	El-Shahaly and El-Sherif, 1991	Ainsworth and Aulicino, 1993	Hudson, 1995	Adib, 2005	Our Data
Neck	9.7%		37%		46.3%
Thoracic spine		70%	80%	40%	27.8%
Lower Back	24.6%				31.5%
Upper limbs			59%		
Shoulders	21.9%			6%	40.7%
Elbows	21%			9%	22.2%
Wrists					40.7%
Hand/fingers	12.3%	27%			
Hips				9%	27.8%
Lower limbs			57%		
Knees	32.4%			73%	61.1%
Ankles	7%			26%	44.4%
Feet	21%			34%	
Multiple sites (>4)	13.1%				55%

For severe pain, more powerful narcotics may be necessary including morphine. For patients that experience moderate to severe pain at least once per week, it is often suggested they are followed by a pain specialist. Some patients do report relief with dermal patches usually of narcotics or anesthetic (numbing) properties. Use of lidocaine patches, although effective, must be used with caution. It has been noted in many patients that topical anesthetics are poorly effective in keeping local pain control and are rapidly absorbed in EDS-HM patients [Arendt-Nielsen et al., 1990]. High doses of lidocaine absorbed throughout the body can affect the heart causing irregular heart rhythm and sudden death.

Chronic pain syndrome. Musculoskeletal disorders are the most common cause of severe long-term pain and physical disability with decline in the quality of life. Chronic pain in EDS-HM often interferes with routine functions such as: physical activity, sleep, work, social relationships, and sexual activity [Berglund et al., 2003]. Those suffering with chronic pain including moderate to severe flares, often will have sleep disturbance, mood irritability, memory loss, poor cognition, anxiety, and even depression [Figure 4.1].

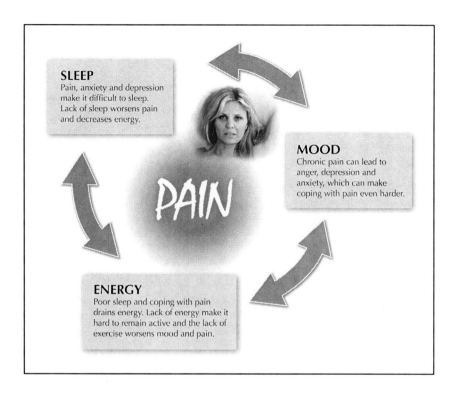

Figure 4.1. The chronic pain cycle.

Pain management in EDS-HM is best viewed as a multidisciplinary approach. Most will encounter healthcare providers who don't believe the pain and/or other symptoms related to hypermobility leaving many affected individuals feeling isolated and confused [Berglund et al., 2000]. Direct pain relief often fails without modifying activities through guided exercises (i.e. physical therapy), addressing sleep disturbance and chronic fatigue, as well as psychological interventions where appropriate.

Recommendations: Treatment of pain is multidisciplinary. Physical therapy is needed in addition to pain management. Appropriate activities and pacing to avoid overuse is a must. Fatigue, depression, and sleep disturbance can all affect the perception of pain and should also be treated at the same time. The goal is to increase endurance (energy level), improvement in mood and anxiety, as well as reduction of pain. Management is lifelong.

Links

Managing Chronic Pain, from the Hypermobility Syndrome Association
http://www.hypermobility.org/chronicpain.php

Pain Control, from the Ehlers-Danlos Support Group
http://www.ehlers-danlos.org/index.php?option=com_content&task=vie
w&id=13&Itemid=9

Pain Management for Benign Joint Hypermobility Syndrome, from the
Hypermobility Syndrome Association
http://www.hypermobility.org/hmspain4.php

Pain & the Hypermobility Syndrome, from the Hypermobility Syndrome
Association
http://www.hypermobility.org/painandhms.php

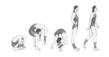

5

—— Use of Medications for Pain ——

Analgesics. Analgesics or "painkillers" are to reduce or get rid of pain. This includes aspirin, acetaminophen (e.g. Tylenol®), tramadol (e.g. Ultram®), and various narcotics including codeine, oxycodone, morphine, hydrocodone, etc. With the exception of aspirin, these painkillers have no anti-inflammatory action. Analgesics are usually prescribed on an as needed basis or taken chronically over a short period of time. Except for aspirin, they can be taken at any time of the day or night, with food or without food, and at the same time as most other drugs. Aspirin and similar products often have stomach side-effects and therefore should always be taken with food. Many feel that painkillers are not dangerous or habit forming provided the maximum dose is not exceeded. Common side-effects include nausea, vomiting, drowsiness, light-headedness, and/or constipation. The dosage needs to be gradually increased for effectiveness while minimizing side-effects.

Non-steroidal anti-inflammatory drugs (NSAIDs). There are many examples of NSAIDs including ibuprofen and naproxen which are the two most common forms. They are often confused with steroids because of their anti-inflammatory properties but they are indeed NOT steroids. NSAIDs are most often taken by mouth but local application (on the skin) at the site of pain is becoming increasingly more popular as it has fewer side-effects. NSAIDs are a form of painkiller but they act primarily by relieving inflammation. Despite EDS-HM being considered a "non-inflammatory" condition, clearly the localized trauma is a form of joint damage and inflammation chronically similar to osteoarthritis. NSAIDs have significant stomach side-effects and should be taken with food. NSAIDs are commonly the first-line of painkillers used in EDS-HM which has the added benefit of being anti-inflammatory. However, because of the stomach side-effects, some healthcare practitioners do not use them routinely for EDS-HM patients [Hunt et al., 2007]. The concurrent use of a proton pump inhibitor or similar anti-acid medication as a stomach protector may be warranted. In addition, NSAIDs can also be used in patch forms that will limit the gastrointestinal side-effects.

Analgesics and NSAIDs.

Usually taking an NSAID plus the occasional painkiller will be sufficient to control the pain in many with EDS-HM but, sometimes, pain manages to breakthrough and appears out of control. A treatment plan should include use of medication(s) at which pain level. Many will take NSAIDs daily, but often will experience breakthrough pain. It is important in controlling acute or chronic pain to act quickly and not wait until the situation is out of control. As soon as the person is aware of the pain worsening, they should follow the management guidelines created along with their healthcare provider in order to gain better control of the pain.

As the pain worsens, if the maximum dose of the NSAID prescribed has not been taken, increase this immediately up to the maximum dosage. It may be important to take additional painkillers to "get ahead" of the pain and bring it under control. This process may take as little as a several hours to several days but eventually, many will re-gain control of their pain. Once achieving this, gradually reduce the NSAID and the painkillers back to the original level as tolerated.

For some people, following these guidelines will not result in the desired effect and pain will continue. In this case, a change in painkiller may be required. They should tell their doctor that they have tried the above regimen without success and a different pain management program should be considered.

Anti-Depressants.

Anti-depressants are occasionally prescribed for pain to help people break the stress-pain-depression cycle [Figure 5.1]. The dose is often smaller than that required to treat depression and, when taken at night, has the added benefit of helping to induce sleep.

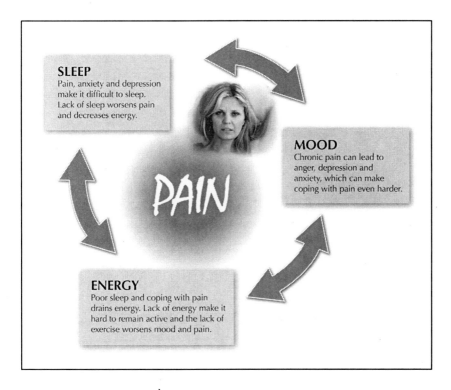

Figure 5.1. The cycle of chronic pain

Recommendations: My choice of first-line therapy is a non-steroidal anti-inflammatory (NSAID) such as ibuprofen or naproxen. Chronic use of an NSAID often requires stomach protective medication as well. Acetaminophen (e.g. Tylenol®) or tramadol (e.g. Ultram®) can be used in addition to the NSAID for further pain control. For more severe pain control, often some form of narcotic, either in combination or alone, is often used. Treatment of severe pain is meant to be short-term and other strategies for pain reduction such as modifications of activities, complementary medicine, coping strategies, and/or physical therapy should be in place.

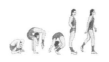

6
——— Physical Therapy ———

The goal of physical therapy and education is the reduction and eventual prevention of pain [Simmonds and Keer, 2008]. Management of joint hypermobility includes any or all of the following [Simmonds and Keer, 2008]:

- Manual therapy

- Posture re-education

- Biofeedback

- Lifting education to reduce pain and strain

- Pacing of activities

- Avoidance of prolonged static (i.e. standing, sitting) postures

- Avoidance of repetitive activities

- Low-impact exercises to maintain and improve fitness

- Education in joint protection

THERAPY

Strengthening. Basic strengthening and guided exercise programs can help to reduce hyperflexibility and increase muscle strength to help prevent further injury. Strengthening exercises, such as dynamic stabilization, are used to promote joint stability by the active, slow tension of the muscles surrounding the joints to strengthen all muscle groups around the joint equally. Education about the proper alignment of the joints and the body in general during all exercise is important as not to stress the joints further. As movements of the arms and legs are stabilized by the trunk, core strengthening is often also necessary to stabilize the trunk and therefore the rest of the body. Exercises that involve high repetition and low weight can also be used to promote endurance. Conditioning activities, such as swimming, walking, and skating, are also helpful to improve joint strength. Inactivity should be avoided. Splints, braces, or taping may be recommended to protect affected joints, particularly unstable joints, during activities.

Joint protection. Exercise should be conducted in very small, controlled range of motion (i.e. mid-range of motion) to protect the joints [Hakim and Grahame, 2003]. Practicing joint protection techniques can help avoid over-stretching the joints and therefore damaging the joints. These may include:

- Avoiding sitting cross-legged with both knees bent ("Indian-style")

- Stop doing "tricks" with your joints to entertain your friends

- Bending the knees very slightly when standing

- Wearing shoes with good arch supports

- Promoting neutral joint alignment as to avoid unusual joint movements thus preventing injury

- Avoiding "popping" or "cracking" joints; in addition to often being annoying to others, this may increase long-term joint damage

Bracing. Supportive splints along with the appropriate footwear can protect joints. Caution needs to be used as prolonged bracing often results in weaker muscles interfering with joint stability/support. Bracing is best used for joint protection during activities but should be used in conjunction with a program to strengthen the particular joint(s) and related muscles.

Stretching. Often in joint hypermobility, some muscle groups will be longer and some shorter to accommodate the increased mobility of the joints. Strengthening and toning along with stretching the shorter (i.e. tighter) muscles provides better joint stabilization. Again, caution is needed to maintain proper joint alignment to avoid further stressing the joint.

Education. Education is probably the most important therapy. It is important to modify ergonomics (positioning while doing activities such as typing) and activities of daily living as to avoid stretching joints past end-range motion. This involves re-education regarding lifting, bending, sitting, standing, as well as activities of daily living. Staying too long in one position often becomes uncomfortable especially in flexed position (such as sitting with the knees flexed). You should move often, stretch, and change positions.

Proprioceptive exercises. Proprioceptive (balancing) exercises may be helpful in reducing pain. These exercises are designed to improve the body's sense of positioning allowing better coordinated movements. Joint proprioception is often impaired in EDS-HM which can result in an unsteady gait (awkward or clumsy walking) and injuries due to falls or joint subluxations/dislocations [Mallik et al., 1994; Hall et al., 1995]. Such therapy is most often guided by a physical therapist and may involve a wobble board, balance stones, or Swiss ball exercises.

Postural training. Good posture reduces stress (wear and tear) placed on joints and therefore pain. It also improves the use of mid-range of motion and overall muscle length. People with EDS-HM often have slumped shoulders due to spinal (backbone) laxity and decreased core strength. Maintaining an upright posture improves pain, joint stress, and your outlook on life. People with EDS-HM also often stand with the knees "backwards" in hyperextension. This puts stress on the joints and continues to keeping the knee ligaments loose. Standing in a neutral or slightly flexed at the knees is recommended. Shoe orthotics (e.g. arch supports) are often necessary to promote better alignment of the ankles, knees, hips, and even the lower back.

Water therapy (hydrotherapy). Exercising in water is low-impact, taking weight off joints thus preventing further injury. It helps slowly build muscle strength. Warm water (83-86°F) relaxes muscles and relieves joint pain. As with any exercise program, caution must be taken into account. For example, if you have shoulder problems, the overhead motions of some swimming strokes may cause further joint damage.

Pilates. The Pilates program focuses on the core postural muscles which help keep the body balanced and which are essential to providing support for the spine. In particular, it teaches awareness of breathing and alignment of the spine, and aims to strengthen the deep torso muscles. This mind-over-body concept is used to encourage improving conscious control over

33

these muscles. Like with any exercise program, without proper instruction, a person with EDS-HM is at a greater chance of injury.

PAIN MANAGEMENT

Transcutaneous electric nerve stimulator (TENS). The TENS unit is hooked up to the skin over particular muscle groups. It sends an electrical signal that stimulates nerves and reduces pain. The electrical currents produced are mild, but can prevent pain messages from being transmitted to the brain. For those with chronic pain, a TENS unit can provide pain relief that lasts several hours. For others, a TENS unit may help reduce the amount of pain medications needed.

SELF-MANAGEMENT

The end-goal of therapy is to sustain muscle strength and coordination in order to better protect the joints. These goals are:

- Reduced pain

- Improved strength

- More energy and stamina in order to carry out daily activities

- Increased ability to cope with stress and anxiety

- Maintain fitness

- Feeling better (improved quality of life)

It is in your best interest if you adapt to a regular exercise routine on your own. Most commonly, these are low-impact to preserve the joints yet give sufficient exercise to tone and strengthen the muscles. Some examples of low impact exercises include:

- Cross-country skiing

- Cycling

- Elliptical machine

- Pilates

- Rollerblading

- Stair stepping

- Swimming

- Tai Chi

- Walking

- Water aerobics

As with any exercise program, consult your healthcare professional before starting. Avoidance of joint hyperextension, such as in cycling, stair stepping, and cross-country skiing, is important in EDS-HM.

Links

Ehlers-Danlos National Foundation
http://www.ednf.org/index.php?option=com_content&task=view&id=15 02&Itemid=88888940

The Hypermobility Syndrome Association
http://www.hypermobility.org/fitness.php

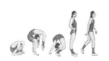

7
—— Additional Therapies ——

Therapeutic exercises, stress management, biofeedback, cognitive-behavioral therapy, and/or nutritional supplements are useful as adjunct treatments as a part of an individual's overall management plan.

Biofeedback. Behavior, thoughts, and feelings profoundly influence your physical health. Patients are usually taught some form of relaxation exercise. Some will learn to identify the events that are associated with their pain(s). They may also be taught how to avoid or cope with these stressful events. Most are encouraged to change their habits avoiding "triggers" for either stress and/or pain. Biofeedback also provides special techniques for gaining self-control so that the patient has the control, not the pain or stress.

Cognitive behavioral therapy (CBT). CBT is a supportive treatment that focuses on the intrusive thoughts associated with depression or anxiety. With the help of the therapist, the person will rationally analyze such thoughts and track patterns of when these thoughts "pop into" their mind. By analyzing such thoughts, patterns are hoped to emerge that can be tested and better responses to such situations are explored. Studies of CBT have demonstrated its usefulness for a wide variety of problems, including mood, anxiety, personality, eating, substance abuse, and psychotic disorders. CBT has been demonstrated to improve sleep outcomes related to chronic pain [Currie et al., 2000].

Diversion therapy. As another form of pain control, diversion therapy is used to occupy the mind as not to fixate on the pain. Many will engross themselves into a favorite hobby or work. Conversation with others is also often very successful in diverting thoughts away from the pain, including group therapy or support groups. However, many use diversion to resume their normal activities even at the cost of more pain and eventual disability.

Heat or cold. Apply either a heating pad/warm pack or cold pack to any painful area and leave in position until the pain is eased. Both heat and cold stimulate blood flow which may ease the pain and minimize swelling. Some will prefer cold initially for its numbing effect. A hot bath or shower may have a similar but more widespread effect.

Massage therapy. Massage therapy provides a relaxing experience by artistic hand strokes on the body to rejuvenate the mind and body and eliminate stress. Physical and psychological stress can induce anger, frustration, and depression that can lead to health problems such as headaches, upset stomach, rashes, insomnia, ulcers, high blood pressure, heart disease, and stroke [Chenot et al., 2007]. Commonly, physical stress induces tense or tight muscles which they themselves can cause pain. Massage therapy not only provides relaxation but increases the circulation of the blood to the skin and muscles promoting recovery.

Relaxation therapy. A form of sleep behavioral therapy involving muscle relaxation, biofeedback, meditation, and breathing techniques aimed at helping the person fall asleep faster and stay asleep longer.

Acupuncture. The oldest healing art in the world. Acupuncture most often involves penetrating the skin with thin, solid, metallic needles that are manipulated by the hands or by electrical stimulation. The aim is to manipulate the energy fields of the body in order to promote balance and healing [Staud, 2007; Wang et al., 2008].

Chiropractic care. The intention of a spinal adjustment is to affect or correct the alignment, motion and/or function of vertebrae (bones of the spine). The effects of spinal adjustment vary depending on the method performed. All techniques have similar effects as other manual therapies, ranging from decreased muscle tension to reduced stress. [Colloca et al., 2003]. Great caution is advised as quick adjustments are potentially harmful due to the ligamentous (joint) laxity.

Prolotherapy. Injection of saline or other substance(s) into the joint space designed to promote a low-level inflammatory response aimed at healing of the surrounding tendons, ligaments, and/or cartilage [Rabago et al., 2005]. Often requires multiple treatments. Its effectiveness in EDS-HM is uncertain at present.

NUTRACEUTICALS

It is important that nutritional supplements (nutraceuticals) be obtained from reputable manufacturers, preferably those that guarantee content and quality manufactured under pharmaceutical control.

Vitamin C. Vitamin C plays an important part in collagen formation leading to stronger tendons, ligaments, and even blood vessels. Vitamin C deficiency also affects wound healing. Maximal improvement of these vitamin C-dependent pathways is approximately 8-50 times the recommended daily allowance (RDA) of 60 mg for adults. Doses of 1500-3000 mg daily are most often used [Mantle et al., 2005].

Glucosamine/chondroitin. Pharmaceutical grade glucosamine (1500 mg per day) and chondroitin (1200 mg per day) has been shown in some studies to reduce pain related to osteoarthritis but not in others. Glucosamine/chondroitin is available as a dietary or nutritional supplement which is not regulated by the Food and Drug Administration (FDA) [Mantle et al., 2005].

Carnitine. Carnitine is a dietary substance important to the body's use of fats in energy production. Carnitine supplements increase the muscle's tolerance to physical exertion and may help prevent exercise-induced muscle fatigue and pain [Mantle et al., 2005].

Co-Enzyme Q10 (CoQ10). CoQ10 is a substance that acts together with natural enzymes of the body in burning of fats and sugars for energy. CoQ10 may also be useful in inhibiting periodontal (gum) disease [Hanioka et al., 1994; Mantle et al., 2005].

Recommendations: These additional therapies are best used in conjunction with the more traditional methods but should work together. Patients should tell their healthcare provider all they do for management of EDS-HM including nutraceuticals and other forms of therapy.

Links

Fibromyalgia/hypermobility syndrome, from the Milwaukee Pain Clinic http://www.milwaukeepainclinic.com/ fibromyalgiaHypermobilitySyndrome.asp

National Center for Complementary and Alternative Medicine http://nccam.nih.gov/

Treatment of Ehlers-Danlos syndrome, from Caring Medical http://www.caringmedical.com/symptoms/condition_detail. asp?condition_id=485

What is CBT, from the National Association of Cognitive-Behavioral Therapist http://www.nacbt.org/whatiscbt.htm

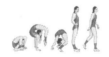

8
——— Sleep Dysfunction ———

"Waking up during the night and not being able to get back asleep at all and taking more than an hour to get back to sleep is a particular problem for me."

"I am constantly rolling from one side to another because it seems the side I am laying on- that hip or side area goes numb, so I turn and lay on the other side until that goes numb. I almost never sleep through the night."

Sleep complaints are frequently reported by patients with EDS-HM. Sleep disturbance was reported in one-third of 125 pediatric patients with generalized hypermobility [Adib et al., 2005]. Many adults with EDS-HM complain of insomnia due to chronic pain but depression, anxiety, and stress are significant factors as well [Mandell et al., 2006] [Figure 8.1]. Many also reported frequent wakenings, difficulty going back to sleep, and

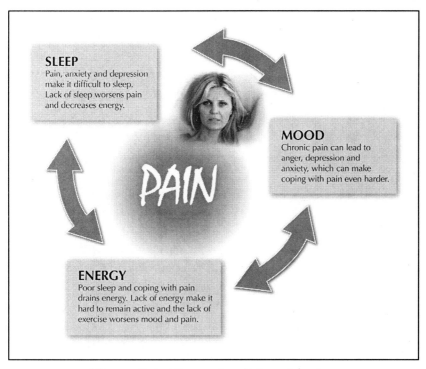

Figure 8.1. The cycle of chronic pain.

41

lack of restful sleep in general. Periodic limb movements (jerking of the legs while asleep) were also found in a significant proportion of EDS-HM patients [Verbraecken et al., 2001; personal observation].

The non-restorative sleep that many experience creates a spiraling downward trend sometimes called the sleep-pain-depression cycle [Figure 8.1]. Chronic insomnia results in higher rates of depression [Benca, 2001]. The overall sleep quality is further reduced in chronic pain patients due to depression that is also seen [Sayar et al., 2002]. Sleep disturbance can also worsen pain, fatigue, and overall quality of life [Kundermann et al., 2004; Ranjbaran et al., 2007]. Thus, pain affects sleep which affects the perception of pain. Non-restorative sleep results in more fatigue, loss of energy, moodiness, and poor memory/impaired thinking- all of which are signs and symptoms of depression. Depression then further interferes with sleep….and the cycle continues.

Sleep dysfunction due to a chronic medical condition does not typically respond to treatment alone of the underlying medical condition such as pain when fatigue, depression, and anxiety often accompany chronic sleep deprivation [Buenaver and Smith, 2007]. Formal sleep evaluation will help in identifying sleep disturbances. Proper sleep hygiene is necessary; which involves: avoiding naps and caffeine; avoiding TV/computer in bedroom; avoiding vigorous exercise immediately before bedtime; keeping a regular bedtime routine and timing. Any sleep disorder should be treated aggressively which will often result in improved energy, better mood, improved pain control, and an overall better quality of life.

Bruxism. Bruxism typically occurs during sleep. It is the grinding or clenching of teeth at night. When it occurs regularly, it may lead to tooth damage, facial/jaw pain, headaches, and/or disturbed sleep. Factors that contribute to bruxism can include stress, anxiety, caffeine, smoking, and alcohol consumption. In EDS-HM, patients who complain of neck pain often have co-existing bruxism [personal observation]. Night splints can be used to protect the teeth and may help with the temporomandibular joint syndrome. Clonazepam, a sedative, may also be of benefit in the more severe cases. In EDS-HM, treatment of the neck pain often improves the associated bruxism.

Joint instability during sleep. Because of the increased muscle tone used to stabilize joints, these joints, when relaxed, may become more unstable during sleep resulting in subluxations or dislocations. The joints most commonly affected are the shoulders, spine, hips, and knees and thus, can lead to acute pain and sleep disturbance. As many with EDS-HM use muscle relaxants or other sedatives, their contribution to the muscular relaxation during sleep is likely of paramount importance and such medications should be used cautiously.

Sleep positioning. Many with EDS-HM often complain of difficulty getting comfortable in bed. Many have used multiple pillows to position and support the different joints often using several pillows ("pillow cocoon"). Many have also tried to change mattresses. Some have preferred the memory foam mattresses as it seems to wrap around the body supporting the joints more evenly. Before spending thousands of dollars on changing mattresses, a physical therapist can help with sleep positions [Figure 8.2]. Additionally, for those more unstable joints, bracing can be used to support these joints during sleep as well.

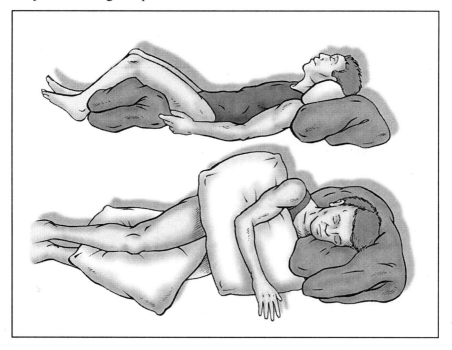

Figure 8.2. Sleep positioning to support the head, neck, shoulders, back, hips, and knees.

Recommendations: An informal sleep evaluation or fatigue assessment can be easily administered. We use short surveys for fatigue (the Brief Fatigue Inventory) and for sleep (Pittsburgh Sleep Quality Index). Often, questions pertaining to refreshing sleep or energy level will identify those with sleep problems. A formal sleep evaluation is recommended to assess for other features of sleep disturbance such as restless legs/periodic limb movements. Proper sleep hygiene needs to be encouraged. Physical therapy can often help with sleep positions but many have improved with just "trial and error". Some will require medication for the various forms of sleep disturbance. Co-morbid conditions such as depression and anxiety should also be addressed.

Links

Bruxism, from the National Sleep Foundation
http://www.sleepfoundation.org/site/apps/nlnet/content.aspx?c=huIXKjM0IxF&b=2450841&ct=3492409

Do some EDS patients suffer with sleep problems?, from the Ehlers-Danlos National Foundation (EDNF)
http://www.ednf.org/index.php?option=com_content&task=view&id=1269&Itemid=88888988

Insomnia, from SleepNet.com
http://www.sleepnet.com/insomnia.html

NIH State-of-the-Science Conference Statement on Manifestations and Management of Chronic Insomnia in Adult,
http://consensus.nih.gov/2005/2005InsomniaSOS026html.htm

Statement on Use of Sleep Medications, from the American Academy of Sleep Medicine
http://www.sleepeducation.com/ArticlePrinterFriendly.aspx?id=194&DType=0

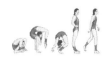

9
——— Shoulder ———

The shoulder and knee are the most common joints that are dislocated among EDS patients [Ainsworth and Aulicino, 1993; Dolan et al., 1997]. Of 34 patients with EDS-HM, Ainsowrth and Aulicino [1993] found that 63% reported recurrent shoulder dislocations and pain.

Multidirectional ligamentous laxity of the shoulder is more often due to generalized ligamentous laxity (hypermobility). This can result in shoulder instability. Shoulder instability in early childhood can lead to the development of a more shallow shoulder joint thereby allowing further instability. Often, the person experiences multiple subluxations of the shoulder feeling as though it goes in and out of the joint. With little trauma, the shoulder may truly dislocate (goes out of the joint and stays out). Such persons are advised to avoid strenuous activities that require throwing, swimming, weightlifting, and gymnastics.

Most patients respond well to physical therapy. Physical therapy is most often used to stabilize the rotator cuff as well as strengthen the deltoid, pectoralis, latissmus, and scapular stabilizer muscles. Open and arthroscopic surgical approaches may be necessary but often fail due to not stabilizing all of the multidirectional ligaments and the inherent ligamentous laxity that remains even after repair [Jerosch and Castro, 1990]. Most patients report immediate relief but often return to instability within 6-24 months [Weinberg et al., 1999]. The initial surgical approach should take into account the inherent ligamentous laxity and "overtightening" of the ligaments should be considered.

Link

Recurrent shoulder instability, Washington University
http://www.orthop.washington.edu/uw/tabID__3376/print__full/
ItemID__254/mid__0/Articles/Default.aspx

10
——— Spine ———

Back/neck pain. Back and neck pain occurs in the vast majority of those with EDS-HM [Dolan et al., 1997; Stanitski et al., 2000]. Low back pain was recognized as one of the earliest features of generalized hypermobility. Howes and Isdale [1971] described a roughly equal number of men and women with low back pain. None of the 59 men demonstrated excessive laxity of the spine or peripheral joints. In contrast, half of the 43 women showed generalized joint laxity. This subset of women also had features that differed from the other women with back pain: it was always in the lower back, they showed excessive curvature of the lower back (lumbar hyperlordosis), the pain usually began in their teens, and that the pain was often experienced only at the extreme range of motion.

Neck pain is also commonly seen in EDS-HM. Such patients complain of pain and muscle tightness. Many are told that these are simple tension headaches due to underlying physical and emotional stress. The pain in the neck can be due to cervical vertebrae (bones of the spine in the neck) slipping excessively passed one another (also called spondylolisthesis) causing irritation and pain. This causes local pain and reaction by the muscles to tighten. Neck pain and headache can contribute to jaw and facial pain. This pain specifically is known to interfere with sleep causing further physical and emotional distress. Some may develop a grinding (crepitus) or popping sensation or noise when moving the neck. If the nerves are also irritated, some may experience numbness, tingling, or weakness particularly of the arms. It is important not only to relax the muscle but also treat the underlying spinal irritation.

Imaging should be considered in all EDS-HM patients with low back and/or neck pain [Chou et al., 2007]. X-ray imaging of the spine in forward flexion, neutral, and backward extension views may demonstrate greater ranges of motion of the spine suggesting instability. Some will also demonstrate that the adjacent bony segments (vertebrae) that may "slip" relative to one another (i.e. spondylolisthesis).

Laxity of the spine can cause a reactive increase in the tone and strength of the surrounding muscle. The chronic overuse of these muscle groups then can lead to muscle spasm and pain. Often, a muscular imbalance develops.

The use of therapeutic muscle stretching (TMS) is of benefit to those muscle groups which have become more dominant, maintaining the stress upon the hypermobile parts of the spine. TMS and postural correction is often of great benefit in restoring the muscle balance and alleviating pain. Treatment typically involves the use of non-steroidal anti-inflammatory medication (NSAIDs) such as ibuprofen or naproxen and rest as a first-line therapy. Muscle relaxants may be necessary but caution is indicated as these can cause a widespread increase in joint instability.

Chiari type I. A large series of patients with Chiari malformation type I were evaluated for connective tissue diseases [Milhorat et al., 2007]. Of 2813 cases, 357 (12.7%) met criteria for EDS. The most distinctive finding among the EDS patients was the presence of fibrous soft tissue (pannus) behind the odontoid process at the top of the spine. The cause of the pannus formation in EDS is unknown but this condition is also seen in traumatic and inflammatory processes. The common features of the various causes of pannus formation include damage to the ligaments that support and limit the atlantoaxial junction; increased movement of the atlantoaxial joint; and recurring subluxation. The surgical procedure for the correction of the Chiari malformation in this group must be altered to protect connective tissue, avoid scarring or adhesions, and to prevent craniocervical instability, a condition when the head becomes unstable or "wobbly" on top of the neck.

Scoliosis. Scoliosis (side to side curvature of the spine) is seen in 30-50% of EDS-HM [Ainsworth and Aulicino, 1993; Stanitski et al., 2000; Adib et al., 2005]. Thoracic kyphosis (also known as postural 'round-back') is also seen in 23.7% of those with EDS-HM [el-Shahaly and el-Sherif, 1991]. Both scoliosis and kyphosis can lead to spinal deformities and back pain, but more often, are not painful and do not require any intervention.

Recommendations: Lower back and/or neck pain should be evaluated for spinal hypermobility as well as disc disease. Treatment is often similar with rest, pain management, and physical therapy. Back pain in the general population is often injury-related; however, the "injury" that has occurred in those with EDS-HM may be everyday activities such as sitting in front of a computer or prolonged driving. Return to such activities should prompt careful assessment of body positioning and use (ergonomics). Occupational therapy or physical therapy can be consulted for ergonomic assessment of the workplace. Often, larger employers may have individuals trained to assess the workplace- contact your Human Resource Department for help.

Links

Chiari and other related disorders, from the Chiari Connection International
http://www.chiariconnectioninternational.com/whatis.php

Hypermobility and Chronic Low Back Pain, from SpineUniverse
http://www.spineuniverse.com/displayarticle.php/article808.html

Info on back pain, from Cure-Back-Pain.org
http://www.cure-back-pain.org/index.html

Spinal Fusion, from the American Academy of Orthopaedic Surgeons
http://orthoinfo.aaos.org/topic.cfm?topic=A00348

Spine and neck, from the American Academy of Orthopaedic Surgeons
http://orthoinfo.aaos.org/menus/spine.cfm

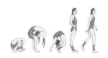

11
———— Wrist/Hand ————

Patients with EDS-HM often have hypermobility of the small joints of the hand as well. This often presents in early childhood with poor handwriting skills or even delayed or poor drawing or coloring. Adib et al. [2005] found that 40% of 125 patients with generalized joint hypermobility had problems with handwriting tasks. Children often adopt an unusual grip that is more comfortable to them but it is often corrected by preschool or kindergarten teachers. As there are multiple bones in the hands, ligaments attached to these bones are lax or loose and thus create a series of looser joints. The muscle of the hands and fingers must work harder to steady the hand when in use. Thus, with increase demand of writing or scribbling, children (and adults) often complain of hand fatigue, muscle cramping, and poor handwriting [Stanitski et al., 2000]. One of the telltale signs is significantly worse handwriting towards the end of a day for a young child.

Recognition of this problem is necessary during school age. Often in grade school, handwriting may be counted against a person's grade. The child may have to rest after writing and may do poorly on timed quizzes or tests because he/she is unable to finish the work due to hand fatigue and/or pain. Occupational and/or physical therapy is almost always of benefit. Often the grip has to be changed in one, if not two, fashions. A thicker writing instrument allows less pressure to be used in order to hold the instrument. This includes having a thicker pen or pencil, or using the pen or pencil with a firm grip that slides over the pen/pencil. Additionally, holding the instrument in a different handgrip may serve better. For instance, holding the pencil between the first finger and thumb uses a lot of muscular strength whereas resting the pencil on the second or even the third finger and using the first finger and thumb to merely guide it, usually takes less muscle strength.

If the symptoms of poor handwriting and easy fatigue of the hand persist, modification of the work is most likely the next most beneficial. This includes additional time on written work, not getting graded based on handwriting, and alternatives to note taking. Use of a laptop, specifically keyboard entry, tends to cause less pain and fatigue and is preferred by many. Additional supportive therapy can involve bracing. Those with significant hand pain especially at the base of the thumb may benefit by a wrist brace with thumb guard which will help support the thumb better and therefore cause less fatigue [Figure 11.1]. In addition, splints which go over the fingers and help stabilize the first and/or second joints of each finger tend to provide some additional benefit. Many individuals are fitted for all ten fingers; however, some elect to wear the digital braces on the thumb and first and second finger only, and only on the dominant

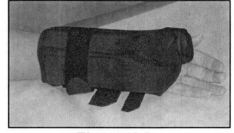

Figure 11.1

hand. Fitting for any type of brace should be done by an occupational therapist familiar with hand/joint laxity. Bracing may be best reserved for those individuals who continue to have finger dislocations. Surgical fusion (arthrodesis) of the bones in the hand is best used in the very severe cases [Ainsworth and Aulicino, 1993].

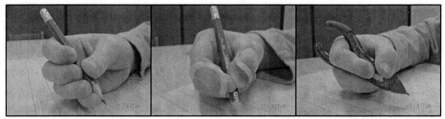

Photos courtesy Mary Flaspohler, OT

Figure 11.2. Abnormal grip adopted by a child with EDS-HM. Improved (i.e. more stable) grip with "figure 8" bracing. Additionally, "ergonomic" pens (e.g. PenAgain®) may also be useful by adapting the grip and muscle pressure used to control the writing instrument.

Nerve compression. Others with EDS-HM complain of carpal tunnel-like symptoms [el-Shahaly and el-Sherif, 1991; Aktas et al., 2008]. It is unclear whether this is carpal tunnel syndrome from overuse or whether laxity of the bones of the wrist creates pain by allowing the nerves to be pinched by the bones causing nerve damage, scarring, and further trapping of the nerve resulting in the pain. Management should begin with a review of activities related to hand use as well as bracing and/or anti-inflammatories. Surgical options should be considered in those with recurrent pain or disability not responsive to the above therapies.

Ulnar nerve entrapment. Ulnar nerve entrapment occurs when the ulnar nerve is compressed at the elbow or, on rarer occasions, at the wrist. Symptoms include numbness, pain, and/or weakness in the 4th (ring finger) and 5th (pinky) fingers of the hand. Treatment involves the use of anti-inflammatories and rest. Avoid leaning or propping the elbow while sitting or working on the computer, for example. Surgical treatment may be necessary in specific cases involving moving of the ulnar nerve at the elbow or releasing the entrapment at the wrist.

Raynaud's phenomenon. The occurrence of Raynaud's phenomenon (discoloration of the fingers with cold or emotional stress) in EDS-HM is controversial. Some authors have reported no difference between EDS-HM and the general population while others have cited an increased occurrence as high as 10%-16% [Al-Rawi et al., 1985; El-Garf et al., 1998]. The cause of Raynaud's in EDS-HM is unknown; however, an autoimmune cause needs to be investigated usually by a rheumatologist.

Recommendations: Close follow up on school-aged children should be done to monitor for poor handwriting and hand fatigue/pain. Occupational therapy evaluation is recommended for any signs of hand fatigue/pain. Often, minimal interventions are necessary such as thicker pens/pencils or a different handgrip. However, some will need more frequent breaks, extended time, shorter assignments, and/or keyboard entry. Bracing often has poor compliance.

Links

Finger splints, from EuroMedical
http://www.euromedical.co.uk/section32/therapy/orthopaedic-supports/finger-splints/

Silver Ring Splints, from the Silver Ring Splint Company
http://www.silverringsplint.com/hyperextension.html

Ulnar nerve entrapment, from the American Academy of Orthopaedic Surgeons
http://orthoinfo.aaos.org/topic.cfm?topic=A00069

12
—— Hip ——

In a series of 125 patients with generalized joint hypermobility, Adib et al. [2005] found that 12% had "clicky" hips at birth and 4.8% with developmental dysplasia of the hip leading to the development of a shallow hip joint ('socket') thereby allowing further instability.

About 5% of EDS patients had congenital (at birth) dislocation of the hips [Badelon, 1990]; however, this occurs more commonly among other EDS types rather than EDS-HM. Congenital dislocation of the hips is not typically seen in EDS-HM but is seen more commonly in the arthrochalasia type of EDS and less so in classic and vascular types of EDS. However, dislocation of the hip beyond the infantile period is common among EDS-HM. Of 34 patients with EDS-HM, Ainsworth and Aulicino [1993] found 40% with recurrent hip dislocations. However, Stanitski et al. [2000] theorized that most reporting hip dislocations were felt to have pain due to the iliotibial band (a muscle) snapping over part of the femur (thigh bone) and not a true dislocation of the hip.

Stable reduction of the hip in EDS is often unsuccessful [Giunta et al., 1999]. However, osteotomy (reforming or reshaping of the bone) to achieve and maintain a stable reduction has been seen in patients with EDS as well as other joint laxity conditions such as Down and Larsen syndromes.

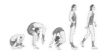

13
——— Knee ———

The knee is the most frequently encountered painful joint in those with hypermobility [Weinberg et al., 1999; Adib et al., 2005; our data]. This is due to chronic ligamentous injury due to overuse as well as pain from the surrounding, supporting muscles and tendons. Acute injury such as knee subluxations, dislocations, and ligamentous tears/ruptures are also more commonly seen. Recurrent patellar (kneecap) instability resulting in dislocations has been seen among 57% of 34 EDS-HM patients [Ainsworth and Aulicino, 1993].

Recurrent patellar dislocation. Dislocation of the kneecap (patella) more often occurs in females (5:1) than males. It is more often seen in their teens or 20's. The earlier the dislocation, the more likely it will recur. Predisposition to recurrent patellar dislocation also includes those with generalized joint laxity (EDS-HM). Patellar dislocation is often evident as it happens with severe pain and a "pop" sound or tearing sensation at the time of dislocation. Often the knee is painful and swollen. The kneecap may be shifted laterally. Manual reduction of the dislocation is often achieved through proper positioning, pain control, and sedation. However, those with recurrent dislocations are often able reduce (i.e. fix) the dislocation with minimal effort. X-rays after the reduction are often necessary to assess for fracture or avulsion. Recurrent dislocations should be managed by strengthening and bracing the quadriceps (a thigh muscle) as indicated to protect the knee. Surgical stabilization procedures are only successful in about half of cases [Weinberg et al., 1999].

Patellofemoral joint syndrome (PFJ). PFJ, also known as the patellofemoral pain syndrome, is associated with abnormal articular (joint) cartilage of the patella, causing pain in the surrounding soft (not bone) tissue, which can lead to true articular cartilage degeneration (arthritis). The most common symptom is a dull ache behind the kneecap, which is often made worse by prolonged sitting ("movie-goer" knee), descending hills or stairs, deep knee bends, and/or repetitive exercises. The joint often has crepitus (grinding noise), locks, or gives way. The malalignment can be seen due to biomechanical problems and/or muscular dysfunction/imbalance. One common biomechanical problem in EDS-HM is the flat foot that results in compensatory internal rotation of the tibia or femur (femoral anteversion). Treatment involves reduction of pain and inflammation (e.g. ice, NSAIDs, and rest) as well as correcting the biomechanics through directed physical exercises such as quadriceps strengthening and/or the use arch supports/orthotics.

Link

Patellofemoral joint syndrome, from the Hong Kong Sports Institute
http://www.hksi.org.hk/hksdb/front/e_pub1_ep2_medicine3_series4.html

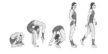

14
—— Foot/Ankle ——

Many persons (43-55%) with hypermobility experience an acquired (or flexible) flat foot and foot pain [el-Shahaly and el-Sherif, 1991; Ainsworth and Aulicino, 1993; Adib et al., 2005]. Typically, such individuals will have an arch to their foot when sitting but when they bear weight (stand) on that same foot [Figure 14.1], the arch will collapse down, being almost fully flat on the floor [Figure 14.2]. This can worsen over time with age and daily activities. Often, the collapse of the arch causes more weight to be borne on the inside of the foot. This is easily demonstrated with the use of "wet" footprints [Figure 14.3]. The result is a slight angulation (deviation) of the foot relative to the ankle, adding additional ankle strain and often pain with prolonged activity [Figure 14.4]. Symptoms of flat feet can also include:

- Your feet tire easily or become painful with prolonged standing.
- Irregular wear patterns on your shoes.
- Walk with toes inward (pigeon-toed) to help keep balance.
- Lower leg pain or weakness.
- Pain on the inside of the ankle.
- Pain in the arch, heel, ankle, or along the outside of the foot.

The alignment of the leg's muscles and bones try to adjust to compensate. The abnormal alignment results in the knees often crowding in or "knock-kneed" (genu valgum). This again creates an imbalance of the muscles supporting the knee and can result in pain and additional instability of the knee. Further, the thigh bones can also rotate, putting additional strain on the hips and the lower back and may be the cause of lower back pain in some with EDS-HM.

Often, the process of the flattened foot does occur with age even without hypermobility. However, as we get older, joints also stiffen. In young children with hypermobility, the flattening of the foot is too quick and allows the collapse of the arch [Figure 14.2]. Most often children are described as being somewhat clumsy, typically falling, or having unusual (awkward) walking or running. This is mostly due to the abnormal alignment of the foot, ankle, and knee. There is some debate though, whether the sense of foot position is also abnormal in patients with hypermobility, also known as proprioception which can also lead to awkward walking [Mallik et al., 1994; Hall et al., 1995].

Foot pain. Many children also complain of "growing pains". This is the relative tightness of the leg muscles that occurs during rapid growth spurts. The pain typically occurs late in the day and usually involves the lower thigh or knee but can affect the foot and ankle as well. This pain can be due to the tight muscles or separately, due to the overuse of the leg muscles compensating for the knee and/or ankle instability. More significant pain may interfere with sleep. Known aggravating activities should be either modified or curtailed totally. There is some benefit with taking NSAIDs such as ibuprofen before the activity. If pain is due to tightened muscles, these muscles may benefit from stretching exercises.

Physical therapy for the foot/ankle. Those with recurrent or chronic pain may require management with the use of a shoe insert or custom-made orthotic which places a device underneath the arch providing additional support. This then changes the dynamics of the foot/ankle relative to the ankle position and can lead to better weight distribution and less stress and therefore less pain. In children, support of the arch may allow the loose muscles and tendons to eventually tighten forming a more normal arch. Some children may require ankle orthoses (braces) which will provide significantly more ankle support; however, at the cost of working the muscles less. It is important for any use of bracing that an ongoing program of muscle strengthening takes place. Some individuals may gain sufficient strength and tightening of the ligaments that such braces may eventually come off; however, many older children and adults will continue to benefit from shoe orthotics.

Physical therapy is indicated for ankle instability or restricted range of motion. Most will require resistance training, reactive neuromuscular training, and proprioceptive training. Resistance training can involve leg press, calf raise, knee extensor, and knee flexor exercises with increasing resistance over time. Reactive neuromuscular training uses resistance tubing to strengthen the ankle. Proprioceptive exercises are designed to promote sense of balance as gauged by joint position "sense" which is thought to be deficient in EDS-HM [Mallik et al., 1994; Hall et al., 1995].

If malalignment of the ankle, knee, and hip do occur, directed physical therapy to rebalance the muscles may also be necessary to correct the knock-kneed deformity, the rotation of the thigh bone (femoral anteversion), as well as hip and lower back pain. It is believed that these altered mechanics resulting in malalignment can significantly wear a joint unevenly and predispose to joint subluxation or true dislocations as well as early-onset arthritis.

In addition to the orthotics and physical therapy, there is some physical therapy exercises designed to increase the strength of the foot muscles. This includes rolling a ball with the feet as well as picking up objects with one's toes. It is thought that strengthening the foot will provide some additional support of the loose ligaments in the foot. However, this is an unproven approach in hypermobility.

Foot/ankle surgery. Surgical approaches to foot pain with hypermobility are often unsuccessful. The more common surgical approach is to stretch a ligament around different bony structures tightening the ankle. However, as this ligament is also hyperlax, it will often again stretch over time. One method, although somewhat controversial, is to fuse some of the bones in the foot, which is called arthrodesis. The foot, much like the hand, is made up of multiple small bones. It is these bones that are allowed to settle, collapsing the foot. The surgical approach is to take two or three of these bones and fuse them together, not allowing them to collapse further. This has minimal effect on overall joint mobility but often can stabilize the hindfoot (heel) and ankle to a much greater degree. Experience with this type of surgical approach is limited and surgery should not be approached lightly.

Other surgical methods are available and may have more beneficial effects for those with EDS-HM. Arthroresis utilizes implantation of small devices between the bones of the foot in the joint spaces that limits but does not eliminate the joint flexibility. This approach is less invasive and less aggressive for the hypermobile foot. Currently, new devices used to replace the hyperlax ligaments have been introduced. These devices would replace that "old, stretched-out" ligament with a new material that would literally act like one of your own ligaments. Much excitement surrounds the prospect of such a surgical approach in EDS-HM and other connective tissue disorders. Caution: these procedures are relatively new and some insurance plans including state insurance providers have considered these approaches as investigational and are not covered.

Although foot pain is predominately related to stretching of the ligaments and nerves due to the collapse of the arch, others experience different types of foot pain. This may be related to an overstretching of the ligaments which can result in tearing of the ligaments or partial detachment of the same ligaments. Partial detachment can create a further unstable joint and may require surgical fixation. Some of the detached bone fragments from torn ligaments can lodge in the joint spaces causing pain. Additionally, as the ligaments are lax, the area between the bones which is normally very narrow can increase. This can allow nearby structures to fall between bones and to get pinched. This includes both nerves and blood vessels creating pain and/or numbness. Therapy for this is similar as for flat feet. However, more serious "pinching" of the nerves or blood vessels may need surgical correction.

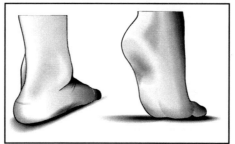

Figure 14.1. The flexible flat foot will collapse upon standing but may appear normal when not bearing weight or when standing.

Figure 14.2. Flattening of the arch as compared to normal.

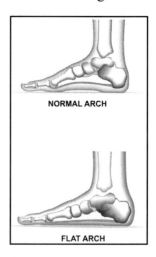

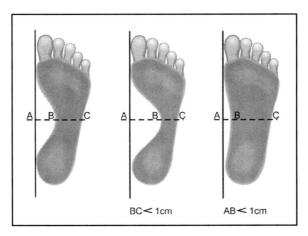

Figure 14.3. To tell if you have flat feet, simply wet your feet then stand on a flat dry surface which will leave an imprint of your foot. Flat feet have a nearly complete imprint (footprint) which can be measured.

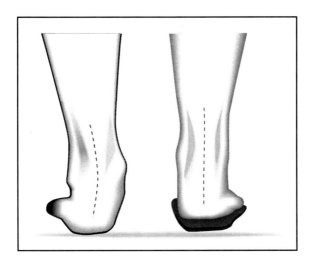

Figure 14.4. The collapse of the arch causes angulation of the ankle placing more weight on the inside of the ankle/foot. A shoe orthotic that supports the heel or the arch can reduce the angulation and allow more equal distribution of weight.

Links

*Adult flatfoot clinical practice guidelines, from the American College
Foot and Ankle Surgeons
http://www.acfas.org/NR/rdonlyres/C312BA90-5BE8-40AD-AFA7-
2CD867862A22/0/AdultFlatfootCPG.pdf*

*Flat feet, from the Mayo Clinic
http://www.mayoclinic.com/health/flatfeet/DS00449*

*Foot & Ankle, from the American Academy of Orthopaedic Surgeons
http://orthoinfo.aaos.org/menus/foot.cfm*

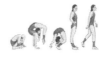

15

Surgery

Surgical outcomes for those with EDS-HM are more variable and typically poorer than those without EDS [Aldridge et al., 2003; Rose et al., 2004]. Surgery for unstable joints due to ligamentous laxity alone fails nearly 50% of the time. However, ligamentous tears or tendon ruptures may occur more frequently in EDS-HM and will often need to be corrected surgically [Goldberg, 1987].

Flat foot (a.k.a. pes planus). Several surgical procedures have been developed for the painful flexible flat foot. Most procedures involve arthrodesis or fusion of one, two, or three of the bones in the hindfoot. Triple arthrodesis is used to stabilize the subtalar and talonavicular joints which increase the stability of the foot. Other procedures combine arthrodesis as well as other techniques such as tendon transfer (relocation). No one procedure has been shown to be more effective than others in all cases but some advocate triple arthrodesis as the preferred approach in cases of generalized joint hypermobility [Ainsworth and Aulicino, 1993; Canale, 1998].

Chronic patellar instability. Recurrent dislocation of the kneecap (patella) occurs in a minority of those with hypermobility but can be very painful and disabling. Initially, physical therapy involving quadriceps isometrics, straight leg raises, and single-plane motion exercises will help stabilize the knee. If the patella continues to be unstable despite rehabilitation, surgery should be considered. In adolescents and young adults, primary ligamentous repair may need to be complemented by bony reconstruction of the joint (osteotomy).

Spinal fusion. Fusion or "welding" of two or more vertebrae (bones) of the spine can be used to treat injuries, disc herniation, abnormal curvature of the spine, or a weak/unstable spine- any of which can be seen more commonly in EDS-HM. Fusing together two or more vertebrae together will help stabilize the spine. The spinal fusion eliminates motion between vertebral segments which can be a significant source of pain in some. This will take away some spinal flexibility but as most spinal fusions involve only small segments, they do not limit motion very much. This approach must be done cautiously as some studies have shown increased hypermobility of the segment adjacent to the fused area [Park et al., 2007; Spakauskas et al., 2007]. However, another study showed no clinical differences up to five years after fusion in the lumbar spine [Axelsson et al., 2007]. In our experience, a few EDS patients that have undergone segmental spinal fusion may develop areas of instability including spondylolisthesis that are not adjacent to the fused area [Nematbakhsh and Crawford, 2004; personal observation]. Whether or not this may represent multiple areas of instability already existing or progressive instability due to additional stress placed on the area from the spinal fusion is not known currently. Although symptomatic relief is almost always seen at least initially, awareness of this possible complication in the future is suggested.

Wound healing and infections. More typically, poor wound healing with suture failure is seen in the classic and vascular types of EDS. Wound complications are typically low in EDS-HM but may be higher than in the general population [Weinberg et al., 1999]. In some patients, the surgical wound will heal without a problem but gradually separate over time due to the weakness of the scar tissue.

Links

Spinal fusion, from the American Academy of Orthopaedic Surgeons
http://orthoinfo.aaos.org/topic.cfm?topic=A00348

Spine & Neck, from the American Academy of Orthopaedic Surgeons
http://orthoinfo.aaos.org/menus/spine.cfm

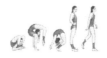

16
——— The Heart ———

Aortic dilatation. As connective tissue contributes to the structures and support of many organs, it is also commonly found in the valves of the heart as well as the supporting structure (walls) of the major blood vessels. The vascular form of EDS is characterized by weak arterial walls, which can cause them to stretch and eventually rupture (break). Although a few cases of classic and hypermobile EDS have been previously described with concerns of aortic rupture (the great vessel coming off of the heart providing blood to the rest of the body), it is not widely accepted that these reports truly represent patients with classic or hypermobile EDS and therefore, may have been confused with the vascular type or another connective tissue disease.

The aorta in both classic and hypermobile EDS tends to be weaker and often is stretched slightly under pressure from the heart. Aortic compliance (how much it stretches) in five individuals with classic EDS was elevated suggesting that the aorta is able to stretch further but the data for four individuals with EDS-HM was mixed [Child et al., 1981]. Much like the joints, the arterial walls also stiffen over time such that nearly one-third of children will have slight dilation of the aorta but as they become adults, this number is significantly less, approximately 15% to 20% [Wenstrup et al., 2002]. Long term studies are needed to evaluate for additional consequences later in life and are currently underway. Our preliminary studies have shown no patients having significant consequences due to this dilatation of the aorta such as aortic rupture and/or heart valvular problems [personal observation].

Mitral valve prolapse. A high incidence of mitral valve prolapse (MVP) was found in patients with EDS in earlier studies [Grahame et al., 1981; Handler et al., 1985]. However, with the use of more current methods and stricter criteria for the diagnosis of MVP, the incidence among EDS patients, including those with defined hypermobility syndrome, was the same as the control (i.e. general) population [Dolan et al., 1997].

Palpitations/tachycardia. Abnormal heart rhythm based on electrocardiograms (ECGs) has been seen more consistently among hypermobile subjects than controls [Grahame et al., 1981]. Palpitations (a forceful often rapid heart rate) occur more commonly in generalized joint hypermobility possibly related to a dysfunction of the autonomic nervous system (the nerves that control breathing and heart rate) [Gazit Y et al., 2003]. One-third to nearly one-half of EDS-HM patients reported atypical chest pain [Ainsworth and Aulicino, 1993; Dolan et al., 1997]. Most also reported palpitations while some were previously diagnosed with tachycardia (fast heart rate) at much higher incidences than in controls.

Orthostatic hypotension and postural orthostatic tachycardia syndrome (POTS). Orthostatic hypotension, also known as postural hypotension, refers to a lower than expected blood pressure upon changing positions such as from lying to standing. Symptoms often include lightheadedness, dizziness, and/or fainting. POTS is defined as a heart rate increase greater than thirty beats per minute from supine (laying on one's back) to standing. Symptoms of POTS also include weakness, dizziness, lightheadedness, blurred vision, and loss of consciousness (fainting). Many will report rapid heart rate (tachycardia), anxiety, and tremulousness (feeling of nervousness). Some will report gastrointestinal complaints such as nausea, cramps, bloating, and constipation. Both orthostatic hypotension and POTS are typically seen more frequently among the elderly but have been reported to be associated with joint hypermobility in younger patients.

Researchers at the National Institutes of Health studied the prevalence of POTS among 61 consecutive patients with hypermobile and classical forms of EDS. Thirty eight percent (23/61) of the subjects met criteria for POTS. The condition was significantly more common in patients under the age of 25, with 72% of such patients being affected, as compared to 13.9% of persons over the age of 25. The presence of POTS was associated with a reduction in quality of life, including inability to maintain gainful employment or attend school. Low blood pressure is also seen more commonly among EDS-HM patients (personal observation). Such individuals will often describe symptoms with positional changes often without complaining of a fast heart rate (orthostatic hypotension); however, upon formal medical testing (e.g. tilt table testing), such patients often are diagnosed with POTS.

Although the exact cause of POTS in EDS-HM is not known, many factors in EDS may contribute including venous dilatation such as varicose veins, lower blood pressure at rest [Engelbert et al., 2003; Simmonds and Keer, 2008], and autonomic dysfunction [Hakim and Grahame, 2004; Agarwal et al., 2007].

Management includes avoiding such things as dehydration, certain medications (e.g. narcotics, tricyclic antidepressants), and physical activity that may make it worse. Many benefit from increased fluid (i.e. water) and salt intake. Raising the head of the bed by 15-20 degrees (4-6 inches) and compression stockings may provide benefit in some. Medications such as ibuprofen and certain antidepressants may have side-effects that reduce symptoms. Those more symptomatic may benefit from a mineralocorticoid such as fludrocortisone, which will increase the blood volume.

Recommendations: A baseline echocardiogram with detailed measurements of the aortic root, sinotubular junction, and the ascending aorta should be obtained. In the case of aortic dilatation, such patients are seen for repeat echocardiogram in 6-12 months to determine progression. Few with EDS-HM ever require medical intervention. Many patients are followed yearly or every two years with cardiac examination and echocardiography. Adults over 25 years of age are often no longer followed if no concerns are present. Long-term consequences of the aortic dilatation are not known and a low threshold should be assumed for anyone with EDS-HM and evaluated appropriately.

Links

Orthostatic hypotension, from Dr. Timothy Hain
http://www.dizziness-and-balance.com/disorders/medical/orthostatic.
html

Orthostatic hypotension, from the Mayo Clinic
http://www.mayoclinic.com/health/orthostatic-hypotension/DS00997

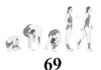

17
—— Dizziness/Light-headedness ——

Presyncopal spells (near-fainting episodes) are common in generalized joint hypermobility [Gazit et al., 2003]. Several theories exist and no single one may be correct for all persons. Those with EDS-HM often have low blood pressure, in addition to an inappropriate blood pressure response (orthostatic intolerance) which has been seen in 78% of those with EDS-HM as compared to 10% of controls [Gazit et al., 2003]. This low blood pressure and the delayed response to changes in position, such as from sitting to standing, may cause one to feel light-headed which often clears within seconds. However, some will actually faint or "pass out". Caution should be taken when ill, with changes in temperature (e.g. from a hot shower to a cold bathroom), and from changing positions from lying to standing.

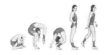

18
———— Headaches ————

Headaches are a common complaint of many individuals in the general population. They can be related to foods, temperature, emotional stress, injury, dehydration, as well as genetic influences. Patients with EDS do suffer with headaches of a multitude variety [Sacheti et al., 1997; Jacome, 1999]. They often experience severe headaches, usually described as migraine-like in quality but may not have the classic symptoms related to sound and light sensitivity. Many complain of headaches related to the neck (tension headaches) which can often affect the forehead as well. Additionally, jaw laxity and temporomandibular joint dysfunction pain can cause significant facial pain which can trigger muscle spasms in the neck as well. Such patients often describe grinding of their teeth (bruxism) in their sleep as well as waking up with dull and sometimes sharp headaches in the mornings.

Recommendations:
- Headaches often respond to typical treatments including mild pain medications such as Tylenol ®, ibuprofen, or Excedrin ®.
- If migraine-like in quality, avoid triggers such as certain foods, stress, poor eating, and dehydration.
- At the onset of a migraine-like headache, encourage plenty of fluids (at least 32 ounces initially) as soon as possible.
- Physical therapy may improve tension headaches, neck pain and/or bruxism.
- Dental (mouth) guards for bruxism protect the teeth but do not prevent the jaw pain.
- Muscle relaxants should be used with great caution as the muscles are compensating for loose joints. Muscle relaxation then can cause further joint instability and some will experience an increase in the number of joint dislocations and therefore pain.
- If headaches are recurring or will not break, see your primary care provider for additional medication(s) or evaluation(s) as appropriate.

19
——— Eyes/Vision ———

Nearsightedness. Nearsightedness (myopia) is a common feature among patients with EDS-HM but it is also common among the general population. Half of EDS-HM patients reported being near-sighted [Ainsworth and Aulicino, 1993] as compared to 50-77% in the adult general population.

Strabismus. Pemberton et al. [1966] noted that 7 of 100 patients with EDS had strabismus and speculated that this was due to the laxity of the tendons of the muscles of the eye. While exacting figures are not available in the literature, strabismus does seem to be encountered more often in patients with EDS and more often refractory to surgical correction than a comparable population [personal observation].

Blue sclerae. A small proportion with generalized joint hypermobility may also have eyes with bluish sclerae [Pemberton et al., 1966; Adib et al., 2005]. In all cases, other syndromes with joint laxity such as osteogenesis imperfecta and Russell-Silver syndrome should be considered in addition to the kyphoscoliotic type of EDS.

Keratoconus. Keratoconus is the alteration of the shape of the cornea (the outer covering of the eye) due to a reduction of the corneal thickness. Patients with the kyphoscoliotic form of EDS can have keratoconus but the incidence among other types of EDS, including EDS-HM, is very rare [McDermott et al., 1998].

Recommendations:
- Baseline ophthalmologic evaluation may be indicated for all those with EDS-HM. Follow up as warranted except in cases of the vascular and kyphoscoliotic forms of EDS.
- Caution with refractive surgery (vision correction). The cornea may be thin in connective tissue disorders. Evaluation before surgery should include corneal mapping to measure the thickness of the cornea BEFORE proceeding to surgery.

Link

Role of collagen in the Eye, EDNF Northern California Branch
http://www.ehlersdanlos.ca/eyes.html

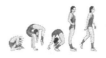

20

——— Jaw and Dental Issues ———

Many patients have unique dental issues commonly seen among hypermobility patients. There is a higher than usual incidence of tooth fracture; periodontal disease; mucosal sensitivity and fragility [Hagberg et al., 2004]; dental caries (tooth decay) [De Coster et al., 2005]; as well as significant jaw pain including temporomandibular joint dysfunction syndrome (TMJ). The gum disease and mucosal fragility are thought to be due to poor connective tissue which acts as a barrier to keep bacteria away from the gumline. This allows the bacteria to penetrate farther, cause additional irritation, and can result in gum disease and tooth loss. A subset of patients will also have significant tooth decay and perhaps brittle teeth. This may represent a subset of EDS with brittle bones, but many patients with weak and/or brittle teeth or excessive cavities do not report significantly increased number of bone fractures. Maintenance of oral health should be aggressive with good hygiene and frequent dental visits. Occasionally oral doxycycline, an antibiotic that helps with periodontal disease, may be used to help prevent further destruction.

EDS-HM is also a concern to many dentists and oral surgeons for prolonged bleeding. This is a feature more typically found in patients with the classic form of EDS which can sometimes be confused with the hypermobile type. Such persons may have prolonged gum bleeding from procedures but this is often controlled without significant consequences and does not require special precautions.

Temporomandibular joint dysfunction (TMJ). The temporomandibular joint opens and closes like a hinge as well as slides forward, backward, and from side to side. During chewing, it sustains an enormous amount of pressure. Many with joint hypermobility complain of pain and jaw "clicking" consistent with TMJ [Buckingham et al., 1991; Ainsworth and Aulicino, 1993]. In EDS-HM, this is mostly due to the excessive laxity of the jaw hinge (joint). This jaw hyperlaxity can cause it to dislocate or to have excessive movement causing irritation. Repeated jaw movements will therefore likely cause greater and greater pain and may eventually lead to arthritis of the jaw.

Symptoms of TMJ can include headaches, tenderness of the muscles, jaw clicking, or locking of the jaw. TMJ may result in facial pain or headaches due to muscle and/or joint irritation. Other symptoms can include pain or stiffness in the neck radiating to the arms, dizziness, earaches or stuffiness in the ears, and disrupted sleep. Those with temporomandibular disorders often report other conditions including chronic fatigue syndrome, sleep disturbance, migraines, and fibromylagia [Hampton, 2008]. Such features are also commonly seen in EDS-HM, and interestingly enough, of 70 patients with TMJ, 38 (54%) met criteria of EDS-HM [Buckingham et al., 1991].

The diagnosis of TMJ is based solely on a person's medical history and on a physical examination. Part of the examination may involve gently pressing on the side of the face or placing the little finger in the person's ear and gently pressing forward while the person opens and closes the jaw. Also, the doctor gently presses on the chewing muscles to detect pain or tenderness and notes whether the jaw slides when the person bites. If hypermobility is the cause, the person generally can open the mouth wider than the breadth of three fingers.

Treatment varies considerably according to the cause. In hypermobility, splint therapy may be required in addition to analgesics (e.g. NSAIDs) to relieve pain. Prevention and treatment of dislocation resulting from hypermobility is to avoid excessive range of motion. For prevention, people often benefit from talking and chewing with a more tightly closed mouth to allow the ligaments of the jaw to rest and shorten (tighten) over time. These individuals also complain of dental procedures causing muscle cramps and pain. This should be openly discussed with your dental health provider and you should take frequent breaks during prolonged dental examination or treatments. Treatment of chronic pain or frequent dislocation often involves physical therapy in addition to the NSAIDs. Deep penetrating heat or friction muscle massage may relax stiff painful muscles as well. Surgery to tighten the ligaments of the temporomandibular joint is rarely necessary to prevent recurrent dislocations.

Gum disease. The oral mucosa, or the tissue lining the mouth, is very fragile, prone to injury and infections as well as particularly vulnerable to sharp objects such as orthodontic appliances (braces) or partial dentures. Mucosal fragility was seen in 74% of EDS patients [De Coster et al., 2005].

Early-onset periodontal disease (gum disease) has been seen in various forms of EDS and for a period, was its own separate type, EDS VIII. Most cases are described in classic EDS but it is not uncommon to find similar early-onset and/or recurrent periodontal disease in EDS-HM [Reichert et al., 1999; personal observation]. Periodontal disease is treated with good oral hygiene including regular dental visits, removal of any substance along the gumline, and antibiotic therapy which may include doxycycline [Perez et al., 2002].

Bruxism. Bruxism typically occurs during sleep. It is the grinding or clenching of teeth at night. When it occurs regularly, it may lead to tooth damage, facial/jaw pain, headaches, and/or disturbed sleep. Factors that contribute to bruxism can include stress, anxiety, caffeine, smoking, and alcohol consumption. Treatment involves physical therapy and at times, sedative medications. Oral splints are sometimes used to protect the teeth but do not prevent the TMJ or associated neck pain.

Dental visits.
- Make sure to discuss your jaw and mouth issues with your dental health provider.
- During prolonged procedures, care must be taken to prevent dislocation of the jaw.
- Take brief breaks every 10 minutes or so.
- Because of the poor local anesthetic effect, many view dental procedures as inflicting pain and thus avoid dental visits altogether [Berglund et al., 2000].
- An unusually rapid migration during orthodontic movement phases was noted in some patients with EDS [Norton and Assael, 1997].
- Because of tissue repair problems in EDS, there may be slow healing after dental extractions, followed by soft tissue scarring.

Links

Bruxism, from the National Sleep Foundation
http://www.sleepfoundation.org/site/apps/nlnet/content.aspx?c=huIXKjM
0IxF&b=2450841&ct=3492409

"Dental Manifestations and Considerations in Treating Patients with
Ehlers-Danlos Syndrome", from the Ehlers-Danlos national Foundation
http://www.ednf.org/index.php?option=com_content&task=view&id=11
95&Itemid=88888988

The TMJ Association, Ltd.
http://www.tmj.org/

TMJ Disorders, from the American Pain Foundation
http://www.painfoundation.org/print.asp?file=documents/doc_043.htm

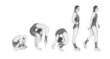

21
—— Breathing/Pulmonary Issues ——

A higher incidence of asthma or asthma-like symptoms has been noted in many small series of patients with joint hypermobility. Morgan et al. [2007] surveyed 126 hypermobility syndrome and 162 EDS subjects. Compared to controls, asthma and atopy (allergy) were more common among both populations as compared to controls. Many more subjects reported dyspnea (difficulty breathing), reduced exercise intolerance, and cough more frequently than controls. In addition, physiologic studies of a subset of subjects revealed further an increase in lung volumes, impaired gas exchange, and an increased tendency to collapse the airway.

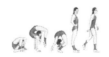

22

Abdominal Pain and Gastrointestinal Issues

Gastrointestinal ("stomach") issues are seen in almost half of those individuals with EDS [Sacheti et al., 1997; Levy et al., 1999]. According to a National Institute of Health study, they found a high occurrence of gastrointestinal manifestations in a group of 90 patients with either hypermobile or classical types of EDS [Levy et al., 1999]. In this group, severe chronic constipation (17%), irritable bowel syndrome (12%), acid reflux or gastroesophageal reflux disease (14%), and/or chronic abdominal pain (22%) were observed at higher levels than in the general population. Additionally, four subjects were found to have delayed stomach emptying or gastroparesis.

Gastroesophageal reflux disease (GERD). The hollow tubes of the stomach and intestines are supported by connective tissue. These tubes are a series of layers involving muscles and connective tissue. The increased laxity of the connective tissue results in more difficulty for the muscles to contract. This results in the inability to close various valves throughout the gastrointestinal tract and difficulty pushing foods along for stooling. Once the stomach is full, it will literally grind the food as the stomach is a very strong muscle. As it contracts, a valve at the beginning and one at the end of the stomach closes keeping the contents within the stomach until fully digested. The muscular valve at the top of the stomach sometimes cannot close sufficiently thus allowing the stomach contents to go up the "food pipe" (esophagus) creating the sensation of heartburn, also known as gastroesophageal reflux.

Many patients complain of frequent problems related to heartburn and require medication. Others have adjusted their lifestyle to eat smaller, more frequent meals with less fat content thus putting less volume in the stomach allowing it to empty faster with less chance of creating heartburn. For those that do suffer heartburn, this often requires maximal therapy with medications such as those known as proton pump inhibitors.

Occasionally, the weakened diaphragm allows the strong contractures of the stomach to penetrate upward into the chest cavity resulting in a hiatal hernia. This further allows stomach contents to go up the food pipe creating heartburn. Hiatal hernias are uncommon except in the more obese patients but are seen in a much higher frequency among patients with EDS [Steinman et al., 1993]. Of those with an unknown cause of their hiatal hernia, generalized hypermobility was found more commonly among adults [Al-Rawi et al., 2004]. A hiatal hernia is often overlooked in patients with EDS (who are typically thin) but it should be considered in those patients with persistent heartburn.

Early satiety. Patients with EDS-HM also suffer from early satiety, this is the sensation of fullness with small meals. It is believed that this is the result of the irritability of the stomach and intestines giving the sensation that one is already full. There is some speculation that this may be related to the autonomic nervous system, the nerve system that control baseline functions such as the heart and breathing [Gazit et al., 2003]. Most of those affected adapt by eating smaller, more frequent meals. Early satiety and delayed gastric emptying may be worsened with opiate use to control pain [Levy, 2007].

Dyspepsia. Abdominal pain, early satiety (sense of fullness), and nausea after eating are often encountered by patients with both the hypermobility and classic type of EDS. These symptoms, referred to as dyspepsia, can co-exist with gastroesophageal reflux disease as well as irritable bowel syndrome. Dyspepsia may be caused by a combination of one or more gastrointestinal issues such as the use of nonsteroidal anti-inflammatory medications (NSAIDs), gastroesophageal reflux disease, ulcers, and esophageal dysmotility among many [Lacy and Cash, 2008]. Dietary modification of avoiding high-fat meals and eating more frequent smaller meals provides some relief. Treatment with medications such as proton pump inhibitors as well as antidepressant/anti-anxiety agents often show some benefit.

Irritable bowel syndrome (IBS). IBS is the abnormal movement of stool which may consist of diarrhea, constipation, or a mixture of diarrhea and constipation. IBS is common in the general population and is related to a number of disorders due to chronic stress; however, the majority of those affected with IBS suffer from the diarrheal component. In EDS-HM, patients often suffer from a constipation-dominant form likely attributed

84

to the weakness of the collagen (a type of connective tissue) in the bowel wall or the autonomic dysfunction that may lead to the inability to pass or push food along [Engelbert et al., 2003; Gazit et al., 2003; Bird, 2007]. This is treated very typically by the patients themselves, adopting regular bowel habits, increasing hydration (water) and fiber as well as eating smaller meals. Few require medication (e.g. amitriptyline [Rajagopalan et al., 1998]). However, in some cases, the IBS symptoms do interfere with social and/or work activities. Therapy for IBS is no different than that of the general population. However, successful treatment is often poor with medication alone and patients must undergo dietary changes and regular bowel habits. As with any chronic medical condition, the psychological and social factors in IBS should also be addressed [Hyams, 2004].

Diverticuli. Diverticuli of the intestines are small pockets in the intestinal walls. The little pocket does not allow the intestinal contents to empty completely and can cause pain as well as infection called diverticulitis. This is far more common in the classic form of EDS than it is in EDS-HM, but as mild classic EDS can be easily confused with EDS-HM, patients described as having hypermobile EDS should be considered at risk for diverticuli if symptoms are appropriate.

Rectal prolapse. Rectal prolapse, the herniation of the large intestine through the anal opening (butthole), occurs more commonly in classic EDS and may be an initial symptom for young children. This is more often seen along with constipation. Many patients report recurrent rectal prolapse which is often described as painless but may require manual manipulation to restore the hernia. Surgical fixation has a higher than normal incidence of failure (i.e. recurrence of the prolapse).

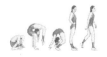

23
——— Pregnancy ———

Most of the medical literature on this subject is based on reports of individual cases and a few series of multiple patients. The medical literature is also often confusing as many publications do not differ between the various types of EDS and their related pregnancy complications [Hordnes, 1994; Volkov et al., 2007]. The pregnancy complications in EDS-HM type are not significant or serious and do not warrant high risk follow up [Morales-Rosello et al., 1997; Golfier et al., 2001; Volkov et al., 2007]. The following is based on the medical literature and expert opinion.

Possible complications:
- A higher occurrence of cervical incompetence is seen in EDS but prophylactic cerclage (cervical stitch) is not indicated for EDS alone [Volkov et al., 2007] but only in the context of true cervical incompetence. Ultrasound for cervical length should be considered at 16-20 weeks gestation.
- Increased joint laxity often occurs more typically in late pregnancy [Calguneri et al., 1982; Golfier et al., 2001; Marnach et al., 2003].
    - o 61% of EDS-HM stated that they had significant increase in joint laxity during pregnancy [Ainsworth and Aulicino, 1993].
- Worsening of symptoms related to postural orthostatic tachycardia (POTS) or neurocardiogenic syncope such as light-headedness, dizziness, or fainting.
- Pelvic pain and hip dislocation occurred more often due to increased weight-bearing and joint laxity [Taylor et al., 1981].
    - o Pelvic pain and instability necessitated the use of a pelvic belt, crutches, and/or bedrest in 26% of women affected by all types of EDS, the majority being EDS-HM [Lind et al., 2002].
- Perineal tears and wound breakdown (dehiscence) is not usually a part of EDS-HM but is more often seen in classical EDS.
- Excessive bleeding during delivery or shortly thereafter has been described in EDS but it is not more common in EDS-HM than in the general population [Morales-Rosello et al., 1997; Lind et al., 2002].

- Risk of prolapse of the rectum, bladder, vagina, and/or uterus during pregnancy, at delivery, or soon afterwards.
- Slightly higher incidence of miscarriage or spontaneous abortion.
  - Among a group of EDS patients from the Ehlers-Danlos National Foundation, 40 of 138 (23.1%) pregnancies of 68 women ended in spontaneous abortion which is higher than the general population [Sorokin et al., 1994].

In the infant:
- Increased risk of premature rupture of the fetal membranes (PROM) which is thought to be a consequence of weakened connective tissue in an affected infant [Kiiholma et al., 1984]. This can led to premature labor and premature delivery as well [Morales-Rosello et al., 1997].
  - In the cases of preterm delivery, the majority was preceded by PROM [Lind et al., 2002].
  - PROM occurred in at least one pregnancy in 26% of those women affected with EDS-HM [Ainsworth and Aulicino, 1993].
  - Among a group of EDS patients from the Ehlers-Danlos National Foundation, 22 of 95 (23.1%) pregnancies from 68 women were preterm deliveries (before 37 weeks gestation) [Sorokin et al., 1994].
- The infant may be small for age [Kiiholma et al., 1984; Sorokin et al., 1994].
- Caution must be used in manual, forcep, or vacuum extraction of the infant at delivery as the excessive joint laxity in an affected infant has caused stretching of the nerves in the arms and legs leading to temporary, and sometimes permanent, nerve damage.
- Some affected infants (13%) are notably lax at birth and often described as having "floppy baby syndrome" [Lind et al., 2002].
- Abnormal presentation of the fetus (breech) occurred among 12% of pregnancies in affected women (all types of EDS) as compared to controls- highest being 19% in EDS-HM [Lind et al., 2002].

24
——— Genitourinary Complications ———

Complications of hypermobility in EDS-HM include a weakened pelvic floor that can result in prolapse ("falling out") of the urogenital organs such as the bladder, vagina, and uterus. In addition, many females with EDS-HM also report dyspareunia (pain during sexual intercourse), dysmenorrhea (painful periods), and menorrhagia (heavy flow).

Periods/menstrual flow. The painful period is thought to be due to muscle contractions occurring with greater force given the loose connective tissue. This intense muscle contraction (cramping) is often at least partially relieved by mild to moderate pain medications. However, for those with recurrent menstrual pain, many will benefit from oral contraceptive use.

Menorrhagia has been seen in 26% of females with EDS-HM [Ainsworth and Aulicino, 1993]. These heavy periods have been attributed to prolonged bleeding which is occasionally seen in EDS; however, this has often been a controversial point. It is considered more likely in the classic form of EDS than in the hypermobile form, but as previously stated, the mild classic form may be similar in characteristics as EDS-HM. The exact cause remains unknown. Treatment is often oral contraceptive use.

Genitourinary prolapse. The pelvic floor which helps holds up the bladder and uterus often can be stretched with age, being overweight, repeated heavy lifting, pregnancy, and/or a connective tissue disease such as EDS-HM. The most common symptom of pelvic floor prolapse is a sensation of pelvic pressure or heaviness as well as protrusion ("falling out") of the pelvic organs through the vaginal vault. These sensations are often improved with rest but worsen throughout the day and with physical activity. Many will develop stress urinary incontinence (urine leaking) with coughing or sneezing.

Genitourinary prolapse is seen more commonly among women with generalized hypermobility [Al-Rawi et al., 1982; Norton et al., 1995]. Uterine prolapse was also seen in 26 of 66 (39.4%) women with EDS-HM who were 19 years or older [el-Shahaly and el-Sherif, 1991]. The pelvic

89

floor weakens with age or pressure and eventually stretches to become "loose" often in early adulthood. Typically, this weakening starts to occur after the first or second pregnancy in EDS-HM whereas it is often much later in the general population. Since the pelvic floor weakens over time, Kegel exercises are particularly important after pregnancy to strengthen the pelvic floor in EDS-HM. Avoidance of further strain is also recommended. Shariati et al. [2008] demonstrated that a high fiber diet for constipation improved symptoms of pelvic floor disorders including genitourinary prolapse.

Stress urinary incontinence. Stress incontinence is the result of a weakened control of the bladder outlet. Women may have stress incontinence if they have urine leakage during one of the following:
- Coughing
- Sneezing
- Laughing
- Standing up
- Lifting
- Exercising

Generalized hypermobility was seen more often among 105 women with urinary stress incontinence as compared to controls [Karan et al., 2004]. Similarly, urinary incontinence was seen in ~60% of women with EDS-HM [Iosif et al., 1988; McIntosh et al., 1995]. In EDS-HM, this is thought to be due to a weakened (stretched-out) pelvic floor which supports the bladder neck (outlet). Women with EDS-HM often have weak pelvic floors resulting in the stress incontinence earlier in life, often only after their first or second pregnancy. This looseness is often referred to as hypermobility of the bladder neck. However, the determination of hypermobility at the bladder neck is subjective.

Symptoms may progress over time. Worsening symptoms include spontaneous urination with little effort, bladder spasms, or herniation ("falling out") of the bladder or vagina. It is also important to recognize that urinary incontinence may be accompanied by anal incontinence (uncontrolled stooling).

Management of stress incontinence depends on severity. Pelvic floor exercises (e.g. Kegel exercises) are recommended for mild or moderate incontinence. The use of duloxetine, or similar medication, has also been shown to be effective for stress urinary incontinence of mild or moderate severity but have significant side-effects such as nausea, dry mouth, constipation, and headaches. For moderate incontinence, a pessary (a plastic device that helps support the bladder and uterus) is often used. For severe incontinence, surgical correction is most often recommended. There are several surgical approaches, each has its own merits and depends largely on the surgeon's experience and the patient's expectations. Any one of the sling procedures is probably the most successful in addressing the pelvic floor prolapse due to inherent loose connective tissue.

Dyspareunia. Painful sexual intercourse (dyspareunia) has been found in 57% of sexually-active women with EDS [McIntosh et al., 1995].

Urinary tract infections (UTIs). UTIs were reported more frequently among both boys (6%) and girls (13.2%) as compared to controls (1% and 2-5%, respectively) [Adib et al., 2005].

Link

Female Urinary Stress Incontinence, from the American Urogynecologic Society
http://www.mypelvichealth.org/

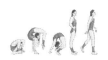

25
—— Hernias ——

Herniation of the abdominal wall or in the pelvic region, specifically the inguinal region (at the junction of the thigh and pelvis) is likely more common in EDS-HM than in the general population [Wynne-Davis, 1979]. Surgical repair often is necessary. Patients with EDS-HM may have successful hernia repair with standard operating practices. However, many individuals with connective tissue diseases can have recurrent hernias even after surgical repair and should be offered repair with a synthetic mesh such as polypropylene that will not stretch unlike the patient's own connective tissue.

Link

Use of mesh to prevent recurrence of hernias, from the Ehlers-Danlos National Foundation
http://www.ednf.org/index.php?option=com_content&task=view&id=13 29&Itemid=88888988

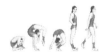

26
—— Skin ——

The skin is soft, often described as velvety or even doughy. The skin may be slightly hyperextensible (stretches more easily) and is best tested at certain sites of the body [Figure 26.1]. However, age, skin care, hydration status, and the amount of subcutaneous fat will affect these skin features. Thus, the skin features are often subjective and there is little standardization in these measures. The evaluation of skin laxity is best performed by someone very familiar with EDS and other connective tissue diseases.

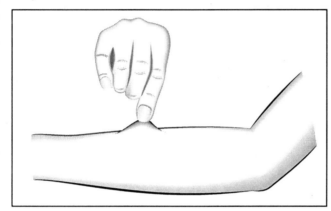

**Figure 26.1.
Stretchiness of the skin is best tested at the mid-forearm.**

Atrophic scars. Mildly atrophic scars (thinned out scars) in places of physical stress such as joints may occur in either the mild classical form of EDS or in EDS-HM.

Easy bruising. Nearly half to three-quarters of EDS-HM patients self-reported easy bruising [Ainsworth and Aulicino, 1993; Dolan et al., 1997; Adib et al., 2005]. Excessive bruising may be more consistent with the classic or vascular forms of EDS rather than EDS-HM. Vitamin C is often given to EDS patients with excessive bruising as 2-4 grams daily for adults or appropriately lower for children.

Varicose veins. Varicose veins were reported in 30-50% of EDS patients [Ainsworth and Aulicino, 1993; Dolan et al., 1997]. Support hosiery can be used to prevent worsening of the varicosities. Surgical treatment has benefited some whereas many complain of the return of varicose veins or the appearance of new ones.

Aging. Age-related changes in the skin are more rapid in EDS and hypermobile patients [Kobayasi, 2006]. Excessive sun exposure can prematurely age skin even more. Those with EDS-HM are advised to wear the appropriate sun block.

Acrocyanosis. Acrocyanosis is the painless constriction of the small blood vessels in the skin of the hands and feet resulting in bluish discoloration and the fingers/hands will often become cold. This has been reported in some patients with EDS but the significance of this is not known.

Wound healing. Slow wound healing was reported in 40% of 34 patients with EDS-HM [Ainsworth and Aulicino, 1993]. Often, no changes in treatment are necessary but larger wounds may need more support (e.g. different stitches, dermal glue) or longer time to heal.

Link

The Skin in Ehlers-Danlos Syndrome, from the Ehlers-Danlos National Foundation
http://www.ednf.org/index.php?option=com_content&task=view&id=13 36&Itemid=88888988

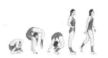

27
───── Local Anesthesia ─────

Connective tissue makes up the substances between cells of our tissues adding supportive (structural) roles as well as various other functions. Drugs absorbed through the skin pass through this connective tissue (known as the extracellular matrix). The rate of passage or dose of the medication is calculated based on a "normal" extracellular matrix. Cutaneous and deep analgesia (numbness induced by medications) was measured in EDS patients and controls [Arendt-Nielsen et al., 1990]. The analgesic effect was more short-lived in EDS patients compared to controls likely due to faster absorption (removal) of the medication. Because of the poor local anesthetic effect, many view dental procedures as inflicting pain and will avoid proper dental care [Berglund et al., 2000]. Caution must be used with lidocaine or other "caines" (e.g. xylocaine, benzocaine) as faster than expected absorption can lead to unwanted side-effects such as a faster heart rate and/or an irregular heart rhythm.

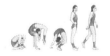

28
—— Muscle ——

Some infants with EDS-HM may be described as "floppy" or with low muscle tone (hypotonia). Low muscle tone often results in joint instability as does ligamentous laxity (hypermobility); thus, the two are difficult to distinguish in the very young. The effect of ligamentous laxity on muscle usually requires additional work and therefore places more strain on the muscle(s) to help stabilize the joint. This can cause muscle fatigue and cramping which has been reported in 77% of 34 patients with EDS-HM [Ainsworth and Aulicino, 1993] as well as pain. Painful muscles are often described as tight and sore. Relaxation of these muscles relieves many of the symptoms. Treatment can include rest, massage, local heat, as well as medications such as muscle relaxants and antidepressants with sedative properties. Caution is advised when using sedatives or muscle relaxants as it is the muscle that is supporting the joint and when relaxed, may cause the joint to become more unstable and even dislocate even in sleep.

29
———— Bone Loss/Osteoporosis ————

Connective tissue, including the ligaments that are hypermobile in EDS-HM, share many of the same properties as bone. Therefore, it is not a surprise to find those with EDS-HM may also have bone affected as well. Fractures among hypermobile patients were more frequent than age-matched controls [Grahame et al., 1981; Dolan et al., 1998]. It is unclear whether this represents weaker bones or more susceptibility to injury especially from falls. However, in a small series of 11 EDS patients, all had decreased bone density (osteopenia and/or osteoporosis) based DEXA scans [Yen et al., 2006]. In addition, Gulbahar et al. [2005] compared 25 women with EDS-HM to 23 age-matched controls and found that the EDS-HM group was 1.8x more likely to have lower bone mass. Similar results were also found by Nijs et al., [2000]. However, Carbone et al. [2000] postulated that the decreased bone density was due to less activity seen in those with EDS-HM than in age-matched controls.

Recommendations: Bone mineral density scans (DEXA) should be done on all adult patients with EDS-HM near the time of diagnosis. Additional DEXA scans should be based on nutritional habits, activities, history of fractures, and any family history of early-onset osteoporosis. Nutritional intervention, physical activity, and medications used to treat low bone mineral density are expected to work the same for those with EDS-HM but no studies have been done to document this.

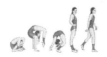

30
———— Osteoarthritis ————

Excessive range of motion of the joint causes stress on the edges of the articular (joint) cartilage which were not "designed" to take this type of physical load [Grahame, 1989]. This chronic overuse of the joint can cause a low-level inflammation and destruction which may lead to developing arthritis.

Generalized joint hypermobility was more commonly seen among women with symptomatic osteoarthritis as compared to a healthy control group of the same age [Scott et al., 1979]. Those with osteoarthritis of the thumb were found to have joint hypermobility significantly more often than a similar, age-matched group [Jonsson and Valtysdottir, 1995]. Treatment is similar, involving avoidance of physical stress on the joint, anti-inflammatory medications, pain control, and physical therapy. Excessive damage to the joint may necessitate joint replacement surgery for some.

31
—— Developmental Delay ——

Children with generalized joint hypermobility often are reported as being clumsy and/or having difficulties during physical activities. Gross motor skills such as sitting, standing, and walking may be slightly delayed [Engelbert et al., 2005; Yen et al., 2006]. Clumsiness and poor coordination are reported frequently which may be due in part to impaired position-sense (proprioception) of the joints [Mallik et al., 1994; Hall et al., 1995]. In a series of 125 patients with EDS-HM, Adib et al. [2005] found that the average age at first walking was 15.0 months, which is slightly delayed. Cognitive (mental) development is not affected. Treatment is needed in only some and usually involves physical therapy and/or braces to help stabilize the joints thus allowing more movement and gradual strengthening of the muscles supporting the joints.

32
——— Fibromyalgia ———

Fibromyalgia (FM) is a condition that commonly affects more women than men and typically in their 30's, 40's, and 50's. Symptoms include pain at particular "trigger" points which are often near joints and represent soft tissue irritation. FM is diagnosed by history and clinical examination using accepted criteria, best performed by a rheumatologist.

FM can either be primary, inherited as a tendency in the family to develop FM, or secondary to other chronic conditions especially autoimmune/ inflammatory conditions such as rheumatoid arthritis. For these types of secondary FM, it is not clear what factors predispose a person to develop FM. Many times the symptoms in secondary FM may overlap with the underlying cause and sometimes will result in an FM-like condition but often respond to similar types of treatment.

Hypermobility and FM are seen together in many patients. Eighteen of 45 (40%) pediatric patients with FM also had hypermobility [Siegel et al., 1998]. Similarly, in a study of 338 children, 43 had generalized joint hypermobility, 21 had FM, and of those, 17 had both [Gedalia et al., 1993]. Hypermobility was also more common among adult women with FM [Hudson et al., 1995; Ofluoglu et al., 2006].

Patients with hypermobility often can develop painful trigger points but may not fulfill full clinical criteria for FM [Bird, 2007]. Many such patients are seen by rheumatologists for chronic pain and are presumptively diagnosed with FM or a FM-like syndrome before being diagnosed with an underlying hypermobility. One major difference is the age of onset. Many patients with hypermobility will be diagnosed with FM-like symptoms in their 30s which tends to be 10 to 20 years prior to the average for the population who actually develop FM. Further, joint hypermobility is often noted in adolescence yet the symptoms of FM often follow many years later.

Symptoms associated with FM include chronic pain, headaches/migraines [Calandre et al., 2007], temporomandibular dysfunction [Calandre et al., 2007], irritable bowel syndrome [Calandre et al., 2007], fatigue, depression, anxiety, and sleep disturbance [Osorio et al., 2006]—all symptoms that are commonly seen among those with hypermobility as well as other chronic pain syndromes. Treatment of FM is very similar to the proposed treatment for hypermobility with only minor differences. Improvement of the underlying hypermobility often improves symptoms of FM and therefore, therapy should be directed at the hypermobility rather than FM per se.

Management of FM has significant overlap with that of EDS-HM including: education, eating healthy, exercise, coping skills, good sleep hygiene, massage, and physical therapy. The major difference is that physical therapy for EDS-HM should concentrate on joint stabilization. Similar medications used in FM include pain medications, anti-inflammatories, muscle relaxants, and antidepressants.

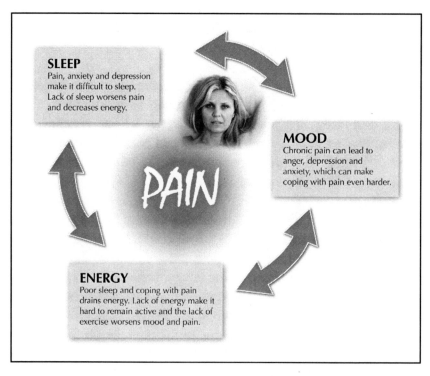

Figure 32.1. The cycle of chronic pain.

Links:

Fibromyalgia, from the Arthritis Research Campaign
http://www.arc.org.uk/arthinfo/patpubs/6013/6013.asp

Fibromyalgia/Hypermobility syndrome, from the Milwaukee
Pain Clinic http://www.milwaukeepainclinic.com/
fibromyalgiaHypermobilitySyndrome.asp

Hypermobility and Fibromyalgia, from the Hypermobility and
Fibromyalgia Support Site
http://anaiis.tripod.com/hmedfm/index.html

Is Hypermobility a Factor in Fibromyalgia?, editorial from the Journal
of Rheumatology
http://www.jrheum.com/abstracts/editorials/200106.html

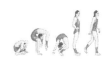

33
———— Restless Legs Syndrome ————

"My legs want to dance/run and they tingle."

"Legs tingle and hurt so bad it feels better to be up walking around than trying to lay in bed to sleep."

Restless legs syndrome, abbreviated RLS, describes the sensation of tingling, "creepy crawlies", pain, and/or numbness that occurs in the legs often late in the day or at night. Many will complain of these symptoms just before bedtime. Often the sensations improve by getting up and walking around.

Minimal diagnostic criteria for RLS [Allen et al., 2003]:
- The urge to move the legs, usually accompanied or caused by an uncomfortable and unpleasant sensation in the leg(s).
- The urge to move or unpleasant sensations begin or worsen during periods of rest or inactivity, such as lying or sitting.
- The urge to move or unpleasant sensations that are partially or totally relieved by movement, such as walking or stretching, for at least as long as the activity continues.
- The urge to move or unpleasant sensations that are worse in the evening or night than during the day or only occur in the evening or night.

RLS is often associated with difficulty initiating sleep, poor sleep maintenance, non-restorative sleep, and excessive daytime sleepiness [Enomoto et al., 2006]. RLS is also often associated with periodic limb movement (PLM), which is the involuntary jerking of the legs during sleep [Lugaresi et al., 1965], as well as anxiety and depression which can also greatly affect sleep [Sevim et al., 2004]. Both RLS and PLM can be primary or secondary due to other conditions. The primary form may be seen among other family members. However, RLS also occurs secondary to chronic pain especially due to musculoskeletal disorders such as arthritis or EDS-HM.

It is my experience that a significant number of individuals with hypermobility, especially those with chronic pain, will have some form of PLM if not RLS. In a small series of 9 patients with EDS, 4 (44%) reported symptoms of RLS and 6 reported a diagnosis of PLM [Verbraecken et al., 2001]. Typically, these individuals will also experience RLS symptoms at an earlier age than what is usually seen in other populations. Treatment should be aimed at both of the underlying hypermobility and RLS. Often, improvement in the musculoskeletal symptoms will also improve but may not be sufficient to abolish the symptoms of RLS/PLM.

Treatments:
- Pain relievers (e.g. ibuprofen)
- Massage
- Local heat or cold
- Relaxation techniques
- Good sleep hygiene
- Exercise

Links

About Restless Legs, from Restless.com
http://www.restlesslegs.com/

Restless Legs Syndrome, an eMedicine article
http://www.emedicine.com/neuro/topic509.htm

Restless Legs Syndrome Fact Sheet, from the National Institute of Neurologic Disorders and Stroke
http://www.ninds.nih.gov/disorders/restless_legs/restless_legs.htm

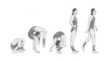

34

——— **Chronic Fatigue Syndrome** ———

"Fatigue is a daily problem."

Chronic fatigue syndrome (CFS) is defined as a profound persistent fatigue lasting longer than six months, causing significant impairment, without a known cause. It is more common among youths and more common among women in general. More than one-third of CFS patients also have depression and/or anxiety [Smith et al., 1991]. Many also report physical symptoms such as nausea (upset stomach), headaches [Smith et al., 1991], chronic pain [Malleson et al., 2001; Meeus et al., 2007], and sleep difficulties (unrefreshing sleep) [Fossey et al., 2004; Unger et al., 2004]

Many of the features of CFS overlap significantly with those of other chronic pain conditions including fibromyalgia and EDS-HM. Several authors have reported a higher occurrence of joint hypermobility among patients with CFS, although this remains controversial.

1. Rowe et al. [1999] described a small series of patients with both CFS and EDS. All patients had generalized joint hypermobility (Beighton score ≥5) and a history of recurrent joint dislocations.

2. Generalized joint hypermobility was seen more commonly among children with CFS [Barron et al., 2002].

3. Significantly more patients (20.6% v. 4.3%) with CFS had generalized joint hypermobility versus healthy sex and age-matched controls [Nijs et al., 2006]. However, Van de Putte [2005] did not find an increase of generalized joint hypermobility among 32 teens with CFS.

Links

Chronic fatigue and EDS, from the Canadian Ehlers-Danlos Association
http://www.ehlersdanlos.ca/fatigue.htm

CFS and Exercise, from the International Association of CFS/ME
http://www.iacfsme.org/CFSandExercise/tabid/103/Default.aspx

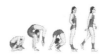

35
——— Coping ———

Initial reactions to the diagnosis of a medical condition are often fear, anger, and/or depression in some and outright denial in others. Most will have encountered healthcare providers who disbelieve the pain and/or other symptoms related to hypermobility [Berglund et al., 2000]. Friends, family, and others may also contribute to the idea that "nothing is wrong with you". For many, getting a diagnosis makes the symptoms "more real" and justifies their pain, feelings, and thoughts about what has been happening to their bodies and how it has affected their lives. Many will feel anger and resentment not only toward medical professionals but the friends and family that did not support them. Others will "grieve" at the loss of their life they wanted to live, feeling the loss of control to the disease. Still some will continue to be in denial supported by the idea that others have reinforced to them that "nothing is wrong" and therefore he/she refuses to believe the diagnosis of the medical expert.

Guilt, anger, denial…all of these are part of a grieving process that nearly everyone goes through. Not everyone grieves in the same way, but still, one must be afforded time and understanding of the "loss of your life the way they wanted to live it". This includes planning on the part of the medical team to allow the patient more control of EDS-HM as well as support for the changes in his/her life that will ultimately occur.

Having a good support system is KEY. Many times, folks can find others with similar conditions or concerns to discuss their thoughts and feelings such as support groups (see Appendix C). Emotional and psychological support is as important in the treatment of this disorder as physical therapy and pain management. It will take time to adjust to having a chronic (long-lasting) disorder. Many with EDS-HM are able to live full, relatively active lives despite their condition.

Fear-avoidance model. The fear-avoidance model is used by some as a mechanism of coping behavior. Uncontrolled thoughts about pain lead to pain-related fear, which, in turn, leads to avoidance of activities [Leeuw et al., 2007]. Depression and disuse may eventually occur, which are associated with decreased pain tolerance and a higher level of disability. This behavior results in anxiety and paranoia. These thoughts and feelings need to be addressed through psychotherapy including cognitive behavioral therapy.

Persistent strategies. Some individuals with chronic pain continue to do the activities that cause pain [Hasenbring et al., 1994]. This can lead to more pain as the muscles are chronically irritated or "hyperactive." Many of these individuals are the "over-achievers" or workaholics. This is a method of distraction from the persistent pain but often can be more damaging in the long term, both physically and emotionally.

Links

A Patient's Experience with Ehlers-Danlos Syndrome, from the American Association of Orthopaedic Surgeons
http://orthoinfo.aaos.org/topic.cfm?topic=A00451

EDSToday
http://www.edstoday.org/index.htm

"Funny, You Don't Look Sick", from the Ehlers-Danlos National Foundation
http://www.ednf.org/index.php?option=com_content&task=view&id=15 13&Itemid=88888988

Living with the hypermobility syndrome, editorial from Rheumatology,
http://rheumatology.oxfordjournals.org/cgi/reprint/40/5/487

Managing the Impact of Pain, from the American Pain Foundation
http://www.painfoundation.org/print.asp?file=documents/doc_014.htm

Strategies for coping in EDS, from University of Washington Orthopedics
http://www.orthop.washington.edu/uw/ehlersdanlos/tabID__3376/ ItemID__32/PageID__8/Articles/Default.aspx

Ways and Means of Coping with Daily Activities, from the Ehlers-Danlos Support Group
http://www.ehlers-danlos.org/everyday.htm

36

Stress, Anxiety, Anger, and Depression

Chronic pain and disability can lead to social avoidance, difficulties with relationships, as well as overall frustration with the medical system [Lumley et al., 1994; Sacheti et al., 1997]. Most of those with EDS-HM encounter healthcare providers who disbelieve the pain and/or other symptoms related to the hypermobility [Lumley et al., 1994; Berglund et al., 2000; Grahame and Bird, 2001]. Yet, pain, fatigue, anxiety, and depression are seen in 91%, 71%, 32%, and 38% of those with EDS-HM respectively [Hakim and Grahame, 2004].

Many with EDS-HM will feel loss of control due to the chronic, disabling nature of the disorder. Fear of pain because of routine activities often results in social avoidance or withdrawal. It is also often difficult to keep a job and to look after a family. Absenteeism from work often creates additional stress and may interfere with job performance, advancement, and financial security including health insurance.

Depression. Depression is a common feature among those with chronic medical conditions occurring in nearly 60%. Similarly, chronic insomnia also results in higher rates of depression [Benca, 2001]. Over half of the adults with EDS-HM reported seeking outpatient psychotherapy often for stress/anxiety or for depression [Lumley et al., 1994]. At least one major depressive episode was seen in more than half of those with adults with hypermobility [Lumley et al., 1994]. Because few physical symptoms are seen in those with EDS-HM, the accompanying depression is sometimes mistaken as the source for the physical complaints including pain, fatigue, and sleeplessness. Many with EDS-HM will report such symptoms as occurring BEFORE signs of depression if a careful history is taken. Nevertheless, once depression or any other psychological feature is present, it too must be addressed as part of the overall management of the patient.

Fear and Anxiety. Panic disorder is the overwhelming and unexpected sense of fear that can cause physical symptoms such as nausea/vomiting, chest pain, rapid heart rate (tachycardia), and difficulty breathing. Panic disorder was found to be highly associated with the joint hypermobility syndrome [Bulbena et al., 1993; Gulsun et al., 2007]. Nearly seventy percent (69.3%) of people with EDS-HM had an anxiety disorder as compared to 22% of controls with other similar conditions [Bulbena et al., 1993]. Conversely, patients with anxiety disorder were over 16 times more likely to have joint laxity than controls [Martin-Santos et al., 1998].

Parenting. As young adults and often parents, those affected with EDS-HM also often fear getting pregnant due to either complications related to EDS-HM or the risk of passing on the trait to the unborn child [Berglund et al., 2000]. Those that have affected children report anger, frustration, and guilt over passing the disorder to their children. They will also fear the future prospects for their children given how EDS-HM has impacted their lives. Many parents will continue to sacrifice for their families and bear the burden of not just the physical pain but the emotional toll as well. It is my experience that many parents will often continue to sacrifice their own care to provide for the family, often at great cost such as permanent disability, loss of job, and loss of the ability to stay involved with the day-to-day activities of their family.

Link

Invisible Disability
www.ragged-edge-mag.com/0301/0301ft1.htm

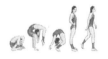

37
History of EDS-HM
———— and the Hypermobility Syndrome ————

Hippocrates is attributed with the first clinical description of joint hypermobility. He observed that the Scythians of the 4th century B.C. as having "flabbiness and atony" such that they were unable to use a bow and arrows because of their unstable (hypermobile) elbows.

Edvard Ehlers in 1901 reported a patient with loose skin, easy bruising, and loose-jointedness. Henri-Alexandre Danlos described another patient with thin, elastic and fragile skin in 1908. It is accepted that these were the first clinical accounts of EDS (classic type) in the English literature; however, Tschernogubow in Russia described a 17 year old in 1891 with thin, velvety, stretchy skin, unusual scarring, and joint hypermobility. In the following years, similar cases were given the name of Ehlers-Danlos syndrome.

Kirk *et al.* (1967) coined the term hypermobility syndrome for those with generalized joint laxity as well as joint complaints that develop repetitive strain (i.e. overuse) injury or symptoms similar to fibromyalgia. Thus, the hypermobility syndrome was reserved for those individuals with joint laxity but without symptoms in other organs and tissues to differentiate from the likes of Marfan syndrome and osteogenesis imperfecta that also include joint laxity in addition to other, serious health issues. The hypermobility syndrome was considered a "benign" disorder (without consequences or concerns) and was subsequently called the Benign Joint Hypermobility Syndrome. However, in the past few decades, other features outside the joints were often also found accompanying generalized joint hypermobility, indicating that this condition was a systemic connective tissue disease.

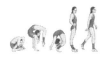

Appendix A
——— Commonly Used Medications ———

Acetaminophen (e.g. Tylenol®)- Mild pain-reliever which can be used in combinations with other types of pain relievers. Daily dosing should not exceed 4000 mg for an adult in a 24 hour period.

Amitriptyline (e.g. Elavil®)- An antidepressant that often provides some level of chronic pain relief, better sleep, and even relieving fibromyalgia-like symptoms.

Antidepressant, tricyclic (multiple brand names)- Used primarily for mood elevation, it is also effective for neurologic pain and mild sedation.

Anti-seizure medications (a.k.a. anticonvulsants)- Although primarily for the use of seizure control, lower doses are also effective in blunting neurological (nerve) pain. They are usually well-tolerated but can cause gastrointestinal side effects and may be sedating as well.

Baclofen (brand name: Lioresal®)- A type of muscle relaxer that also acts to reduce muscle spasms.

Carbamazepine (e.g. Tegretol®)- Primarily used for seizure control, it is also used to treat nerve pain.

Clonazepam (brand name: Klonopin®)- A benzodiazepine medication used to treat anxiety and/or seizures.

COX-2 inhibitors (e.g. Celebrex®)- Anti-inflammatory medications with less stomach upset than traditional non-steroidal anti-inflammatories (NSAIDs) but have equivalent pain-relieving effects; however, this class of medication has been linked to a higher incidence of heart attacks.

Doxycycline (multiple brand names)- An antibiotic that has inhibitory effects against inflammation. Often used for gum disease.

Duloxetine (brand name: Cymbalta®)- A dual reuptake inhibitor of serotonin and norepinephrine (SSNRI) that is safe, tolerable, and an effective antidepressant that also significantly reduces nerve pain as well as anxiety. Duloxetine has also shown effective in treating stress urinary incontinence [Freeman, 2006].

Gabapentin (brand names: Neurontin®, Gabaron®)- Anti-seizure medication, that at lower doses, effectively treats pain of a neurologic origin (neuropathic). Maximal dosing requires titration to a level with little or no side-effects such as sedation or gastrointestinal issues. Maximal dosing should not exceed 1200 mg three times daily.
sleepiness. Low potential for abuse and chemical dependence. Dosing is typically 450

Hypnotics- Class of drugs that induce sleep. May be habit-forming. Includes benzodiazepines, opioids, anti-histamines, and barbiturates.

Ibuprofen (multiple brand names)- Non-steroidal anti-inflammatory medication (NSAID) that acts to relieve pain and fever.

Lidocaine- Often used as a topical (i.e. local) anesthetic for pain relief; however, in EDS, lidocaine (and other "caines") are absorbed more quickly giving less local effect (numbness or pain relief) and may result in unwarranted side-effects such as a rapid heart rate [Arendt-Nielsen et al., 1990].

Losartan (brand name: Cozaar®)- A blood-pressure lowering medication in the class of drugs called angiotensin receptor blockers. It has potential effects on connective tissue that may be useful in the treatment of certain connective tissue disorders.

Metaxalone (brand name: Skelaxin®)- Muscle relaxant that also has some sedative effects.

Muscle relaxants- A type of drug that relaxes the muscles. Useful for muscle pain and/ or strains.

Naproxen (multiple brand names)- A type of nonsteroidal anti-inflammatory pain reliever used to treat mild to moderate pain.

Non-steroidal anti-inflammatories (NSAIDs)- Anti-inflammatory medication effective for mild to moderate pain relief most often associated with musculoskeletal conditions such as arthritis and EDS. Dosing is often limited by stomach upset due to increased stomach acid production which, over time, can produce gastric ulcers.

Nortriptyline (multiple brands)- A tricyclic antidepressant used for mood elevation but has the benefits of relieving neurologic pain and is a mild sedative. Typical dosing ranges from 25-150 mg before bedtime.

Omeprazole (brand names: Prilosec®, Zegerid®)- A proton pump inhibitor that blocks the stomach's production of acid. Used to treat ulcers and gastroesophageal reflux disease (GERD).

Opiates- Includes codeine, morphine, and hydrocodone. Effective pain reducers for both musculoskeletal pain as well as neuropathic pain. Often used in conjunction with acetaminophen for moderate pain. More severe pain often requires stronger opiate dosing. Short-acting forms are available in many formulations for rapid pain-relief whereas longer-acting forms are useful for chronic pain. Opiates can be addictive and should be used under the close supervision of your doctor.

Pregabalin (brand name: Lyrica®)- A neurologically-active medicine that has anti-seizure, anti-anxiety, as well as pain-relief properties. Side-effects include dizziness

mg per day.

Proton pump inhibitors (PPIs)- A class of drugs that block the stomach's production of acid. Used to treat ulcers and gastroesophageal reflux disease (GERD).

Ropinirole (brand name: Requip®)- A drug used to replace the brain chemical dopamine. It is useful in Parkinson disease and restless legs syndrome.

Selective serotonin/norepinephrine reuptake inhibitors (SSNRIs)- Type of antidepressant that works in two different neurologic pathways. Used to treat depression and other mood disorders as well as anxiety, attention-deficit hyperactivity disorder, and obsessive-compulsive disorder.

Tramadol (brand name: Ultram®)- A novel pain reliever that acts similar to morphine but is NOT a narcotic. It produces pain-relief through the central nervous system with an overall effect between codeine and morphine. It has been shown to have relatively few side-effects. Tramadol was shown to be effective in a series of patients with arthritic pain-related sleep disturbance [Kosinski et al., 2007]. It has also been used in children with EDS-HM with good relief and very few side-effects [Brown and Stinson, 2004].

Trazadone (brand name: Desyrel®)- A tricyclic antidepressant used for mood elevation but has the benefits of relieving neurologic pain and is a mild sedative. Usual dosing is 50-300 mg every evening.

NOTE: All brand names are registered trademark(s) of their respective companies.

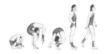

Appendix B
Glossary

Arthrodesis- The surgical fusion of two bones.

Autosomal- Pertaining to a chromosome that is not one of the sex chromosomes.

Autosomal dominant- A trait or disorder that is manifested in an individual when only <u>one</u> of the two copies of a gene is affected. That person has a 50% risk of passing on the genetic trait to each child regardless of the sex of that child.

Autosomal recessive- A trait or disorder in which is manifested in an individual when <u>both</u> copies of a gene are affected.

Behavioral therapy- A type of therapy based on thoughts, beliefs, and behaviors, with the aim of influencing the negative emotions that relate to certain events.

Biofeedback- A treatment technique in which the person is trained to improve his/her health by using signals from the body.

Biopsy- The removal of a sample of tissue for purposes of diagnosis.

Bowel- Another name for the intestine.

Bruxism- Grinding or clenching of the teeth usually during sleep which can cause dental erosion (wearing down the teeth) and pain in the face, jaw, or neck.

Chromosome- The physical structure of DNA.

Chronic fatigue syndrome (CFS)- A profound persistent fatigue lasting longer than six months causing significant impairment without a known cause.

Clinical- Having to do with the examination and treatment of patients.

Collagen- The protein of the skin, tendons, cartilage, bone and connective tissue.

Congenital- Present from birth.

Connective tissue- A material made up of fibers forming a framework and support structure for body tissues and organs.

Diagnosis- The cause or nature of a disease; the identification of any problem.

Dislocation- Displacement of a bone from its normal position.

DNA (<u>d</u>eoxyribo<u>n</u>ucleic <u>a</u>cid)- The molecule that encodes information responsible for structure and function of an organism.

Dominant- A genetic trait that is evident when only one copy of the gene for that trait is present.

Gastroesophageal reflux disease (GERD)- Rising up of the stomach acid into the lower part of the esophagus (food pipe) causing pain (i.e. heartburn).

Gastrointestinal- Relating to the stomach and intestines.

Gene- A segment of DNA that encodes for a specific protein or RNA molecule that has a specific role in the function and structure of an organism.

Genetic- Having to do with genes and genetic information.

Genotype- Refers to the specific version of a particular gene.

Heritable-Genetic element or trait that is capable of being transmitted from parent to child.

Hypermobility (joint)- Also called double-jointedness or hyperlaxity; describes a joint(s) that can move farther than normal.

Inheritance- A genetic trait that is transmitted from parent to child.

Insomnia- Poor quality sleep due to difficulty falling asleep, wakening during the night with difficulty falling back to sleep, waking up too early, or unrefreshing sleep.

Irritable bowel syndrome (IBS)- A disorder most commonly characterized by cramping, abdominal pain, bloating, constipation, and/or diarrhea.

Joint laxity- Also called double-jointedness or joint hypermobility; describes a joint(s) that can move farther than normal.

Kyphoscoliosis- Combination of kyphosis and scoliosis (lateral and posterior curving of the spine).

Ligaments- Tough, fibrous bands that connect bones together across a joint.

Mutation- Any alteration of a gene that differs from its normal state.

Offspring- The child born of a person.

Osteoporosis-A weakening of the bone predisposing to fracture.

Osteotomy- Cutting or reshaping of the bone.

Panic disorder- An overwhelming and unexpected sense of fear that can cause physical symptoms such as nausea/vomiting, chest pain, rapid heart rate, and difficulty breathing.

Pedigree- A diagram of the family depicting the medical history of related individuals.

Periodic limb movements (PLM)- Episodes of repeating muscle movements usually occurring during sleep.

Pessary- A device that is placed into the vagina to support the uterus and/or bladder and rectum from prolapse.

Phenotype- The physical properties of a genetic trait such as blue eyes.

Prolapse- When an organ falls "out of place".

Recessive- A condition that appears only in individuals who have received an abnormal copy of a gene from each parent.

Rectal prolapse- A condition in which the rectum (the end of the large intestine) slips so that it protrudes from the anus.

Recurrence risk- The likelihood of a trait or disorder present in one family member will appear in another family member.

Relaxation therapy- A form of sleep therapy aimed at helping the person fall asleep faster and stay asleep longer.

Restless legs syndrome (RLS)- An uneasy sensation such as burning, prickling, itching, or tingling that causes a strong urge to move your legs most often occurring late in the day or at night.

Rupture- A break or tear.

Scoliosis- Abnormal lateral curving of the spine.

Spine- The column of bone which surrounds and protects the spinal cord. The spine can be categorized according to level of the body: i.e., cervical spine (neck), thoracic spine (upper and middle back), and lumbar spine (lower back).

Spinal fusion- Fusion or "welding" of two or more vertebrae (bones) of the spine used to treat injuries, disc herniation, abnormal curvature of the spin, or a weak/unstable spine.

Spondylolisthesis- Slipping of one vertebra (spinal bone) upon another.

Subluxation- Partial displacement of a joint.

Syncope- Loss of consciousness; fainting.

Syndrome- A set of signs and symptoms that tend to occur together.

Trait- A genetically determined characteristic.

Trauma- An inflicted injury.

Vascular- Relating to the blood vessels of the body.

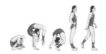

Appendix C
———— Support Groups ————

Ehlers-Danlos National Foundation
3200 Wilshire Blvd.
Suite 1601, South Tower
Los Angeles, California 90010
Phone: (213) 368 -3800
Web: http://www.ednf.org
E-mail: staff@ednf.org

The Canadian Ehlers-Danlos Association
88 De Rose Avenue
Bolton, Ontario
L7E 1A8
Phone: (905) 951-7559 telephone
Web: http://www.ehlersdanlos.ca/
E-mail: ceda@rogers.com

Ehlers-Danlos Support Group [United Kingdom]
P.O. Box 337
Aldershot,
GU12 6WZ, UK
Phone: 01252 690940
Web: http://www.ehlers-danlos.org/

Ehlers-Danlos Syndrome Network C.A.R.E.S., Inc.
P.O. Box 66
Muskego, WI 53150
Phone: (262) 514-2190
Web: http://www.charityadvantage.com/Milwaukee_Ehlers-Danlos_
BranchSQKUQL/Home.asp
E-mail: EDSCARES@aol.com

EDS Today
EDS Today
PO Box 88802
Indianapolis, IN 46208-0802
Phone: (609) 625-3182
Web: http://www.edstoday.org/index.htm

Hypermobility Syndrome Association [United Kingdom]
The Hypermobility Syndrome Association
P.O. Box 1122
Nailsea, Bristol
BS48 2YZ, UK
Phone: 0845 3454465
Web: http://www.hypermobility.org/

American Pain Foundation
201 North Charles Street, Suite 710
Baltimore, Maryland 21201-4111
Phone: (888) 615-7246
Web: http://www.painfoundation.org/

Fibromyalgia Network
PO Box 31750
Tucson, AZ 85751-1750
Phone: 800-853-2929
Web: http://www.fmnetnews.com/

National Institute of Arthritis and Musculoskeletal and Skin Diseases
Web: http://www.niams.nih.gov/

National Marfan Foundation
22 Manhasset Avenue
Port Washington, NY 11050
Phone: (800) 862-7326
Web: http://www.marfan.org/
E-mail: staff@marfan.org

National Organization of Rare Disorders
55 Kenosia Avenue
PO Box 1968
Danbury, CT 06813-1968
Phone: (203) 744-0100
Web: http://www.rarediseases.org/

The RLS Foundation
1610 14th St NW Suite 300 / Rochester, MN 55901
Phone: (507) 287-6465
Web: http://www.rls.org/
E-mail: rlsfoundation@rls.org

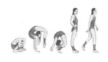

Appendix D
───── References ─────

Abel MD, Carrasco LR (2006). Ehlers-Danlos syndrome: classifications, oral manifestations, and dental considerations. Oral Surg Oral Med Oral Pathol Oral Radiol Endod 102:582-590.

Adib N, Davies K, Grahame R, Woo P, Murray KJ (2005). Joint hypermobility syndrome in childhood. A not so benign multisystem disorder? Rheumatology 44:744-750.

Agnew P (1997). Evaluation of the child with ligamentous laxity. Clin Pod Med Surg 14:117-130.

Agarwal AK, Garg R, Ritch A, Sarkar P (2007). Postural orthostatic tachycardia syndrome. Postgrad Med J 83:478-480.

Ainsworth SR, Aulicino PL (1993). A survey of patients with Ehlers-Danlos syndrome. Clin Orthopaed Rel Res 286:250-256.

Aktas I, Ofluoglu D, Albay T (2008). The relationship between benign joint hypermobility syndrome and carpal tunnel syndrome. Clin Rheumatol.

Aldridge JM, Perry JJ, Osbahr DC, Speer KP (2003). Thermal capsulorraphy of bilateral glenohumeral joints in pediatric patients with Ehlers-Danlos syndrome. Arthroscopy 19:E41.

Allen RP, Picchietti D, Hening WA, Trenkwalder C, Walters AS, Montplaisi J (2003). Restless legs syndrome: diagnostic criteria, special considerations, and epidemiology. A report from the restless legs syndrome diagnosis and epidemiology workshop at the National Institutes of Health. Sleep Med 4:101-119.

Altman RD (2004). A rationale for combining acetaminophen and NSAIDs for mild-to-moderate pain. Clin Exp Rheumatol 22:110-117.

Al-Rawi ZA, Al-Aszawi AJ, Al-Chalabi T (1985). Joint hypermobility among university students in Iraq. Br J Rheumatol 24:326-331.

Al-Rawi ZS, Al-Dubaikel KY, Al-Sikafi H (2004). Joint mobility in people with hiatus hernia. Rheumatology 43:574-576.

Arendt-Nielsen L, Kaalund S, Bjerring P, Hogsaa B (1990). Insufficient effect of local analgesics in Ehlers Danlos type III patients (connective tissue disorder). Acta Anaesthesiol Scand 34:358-361.

Atalla A, Page I (1988). Ehlers-Danlos syndrome type III in pregnancy. Obstet Gynecol 71:508-509.

Axelsson P, Johnsson R, Stromqvist B (2007). Adjacent segment hypermobility after lumbar spine fusion: no association with progressive degeneration of the segment 5 years after surgery. Acta Orthop 78:834-839.

Badelon O, Bensahel H, Csukonyi Z, Chaumien JP (1990). Congenital dislocation of the hip in Ehlers-Danlos syndrome. Clin Orthop Relat Res 255:138-143.

Barron DF, Cohen BA, Geraghty MT, Violand R, Rowe PC (2002). Joint hypermobility is more common in children with chronic fatigue syndrome than in healthy controls. J Pediatr 141:421-425.

Beasley LS, Vidal AF (2004). Traumatic patellar dislocation in children and adolescents: treatment update and literature review. Curr Opin Pediatr 16:29-36.

Beighton P (1969). Obstetric aspects of the Ehlers-Danlos syndrome. J Obstet Gynaecol Br Commonw 76:97-101.

Beighton P, Solomon L, Soskolne CL (1973). Articular mobility in an African population. Ann Rheum Dis 32:413-418.

Beighton P, De Paepe A, Steinmann B, Tsipouras P, Wenstrup RJ (1998). Ehlers-Danlos syndromes: revised nosology, Villefranche, 1997. Am J Med Genet 77:31-37.

Benca RM (2001). Consequences of insomnia and its therapies. J Clin Psychiatry 62 Suppl 10:33-38.

Berglund B, Nordstrom G, Lutzen K (2000). Living a restricted life with Ehlers-Danlos syndrome. Int J Nurs Stud 37:111-118.

Berglund B, Nordstrom G (2001). Symptoms and functional health status of individuals with Ehlers-Danlos syndrome (EDS). J Clin Rheumatol 7:308-314.

Berglund B, Mattiasson AC, Norstrom G (2003). Acceptance of disability and sense of coherence in individuals with Ehlers-Danlos syndrome. J Clin Nurs 12:770-777.

Berglund B, Nordstrˆm G, Hagberg C, Mattiasson AC (2005). Foot pain and disability in individuals with Ehlers-Danlos syndrome (EDS): impact on daily life activities. Disabil Rehabil 27:164-169.

Bird HA (2007). Joint hypermobility. Musculoskeletal Care 5:4-19.

Bravo JF, Wolff C (2006). Clinical study of hereditary disorders of connective tissues in a Chilean population. Arthrit Rheumat 54:515-523.

Brooks JK, Francis LAP (2006). Postural orthostatic tachycardia syndrome: Dental treatment considerations. J Am Dent Assoc 137:488-493.

Brown SC, Stinson J (2004). Treatment of pediatric chronic pain with tramadol hydrochloride: siblings with Ehlers-Danlos syndrome - Hypermobility type. Pain Res Manag 9:209-211.

Buchwald D, Pearlman T, Umali J, Schmaling K, Katon W (1996). Functional status in patients with chronic fatigue syndrome, other fatiguing illnesses, and healthy individuals. Am J Med 171:364-370.

Buckingham RB, Braun T, Harinstein DA, Oral K, Bauman D, Bartynski W, Killian PJ, Bidula LP (1991). Temporomandibular joint dysfunction syndrome: a close association with systemic joint laxity (the hypermobility joint syndrome). Oral Surg Oral Med Oral Pathol 72:514-519.

Buenaver LF, Smith MT (2007). Sleep in rheumatic diseases and other painful conditions. Curr Treat Options Neurol 9:325-336.

Bulbena A, Duro JC, Porta M, Martin-Santos R, Mateo A, Molina L, Vallescar R, Vallejo J (1993). Anxiety disorders in the joint hypermobility syndrome. Psychiatry Res 46:59-68.

Bump RC, Voss S, Beardsworth A, Manning M, Zhao YD, Chen W (2008). Long-term efficacy of duloxetine in women with stress urinary incontinence. BJU Int 102: 214-218.

Burks JB, DeHeer PA (2004). Triple arthrodesis. Clin Podiatr Med Surg 21:203-226.

Calandre EP, Hidalgo J, Rico-Villademoros F (2007). Use of ziprasidone in patients with fibromylagia: a case series. Rheumatol Int 27:473-476.

Calguneri M, Bird HA, Wright V (1982). Changes in joint laxity occurring during pregnancy. Ann Rheum Dis 41:126-128.

Cameron JA (1993). Corneal abnormalities in Ehlers-Danlos syndrome type VI. Cornea 12:54-59.

Canale ST (1998). "Campbell's Operative Orthopaedics", vol 2. Mosby, St. Louis.

Carbone L, Tylavsky FA, Bush AJ, Koo W, Orwoll E, Cheng S (2000). Bone density in Ehlers-Danlos syndrome. Osteoporos Int 11:388-392.

Carley ME, Schaffer J (2000). Urinary incontinence and pelvic organ prolapse in women with Marfan or Ehlers Danlos syndrome. Am J Obstet Gynecol 182:1021-1023.

133

Ceccolini E. Ehlers-Danlos syndrome. http://www.emedicine.com/derm/topic696.htm

Chenot JF, Becker A, Leonhardt C, Keller S, Donner-Banzhoff N, Baum E, Pfingsten M, Hildebrandt J, Basler HD, Kochen MM (2007). Use of complementary alternative medicine for low back pain consulting in general practice: a cohort study. BMC Complement Altern Med 7:42.

Child AH, Dorrance DE, Jay B, Pope FM, Jones RB, Gosling RG (1981). Aortic compliance in connective tissue disorders affecting the eye. Ophthalmic Paediatrics and Genetics 1:59-76.

Chou R, Qaseem A, Snow V, Casey D, Cross JT, Shekelle P, Owens DK (2007). Diagnosis and treatment of low back pain: a joint clinical practice guideline from the American College of Physicians and the American Pain Society. Ann Intern Med 147:478-491.

Colloca CJ, Polkinghorn BS (2003). Chiropractic management of Ehlers-Danlos syndrome: a report of two cases. J Manipulative Physiol Ther 26:448-459.

Currie SR, Wilson KG, Pontefract AJ, deLaplante L (2000). Cognitive-behavioral treatment of insomnia secondary to chronic pain. J Consult Clin Psychol 68:407-416.

De Coster PJ, Martens LC, Van den Berghe L (2004). Prevalence of temporomandibular joint dysfunction in Ehlers-Danlos syndromes. Orthod Craniofac Res 7:237-240.

De Coster PJ, Martens LC, De Paepe A (2005). Oral health in prevalent types of Ehlers-Danlos syndromes. J Oral Pathol Med 34:298-307.

De Coster PJ, Van den Berghe LI, Martens LC (2005). Generalized joint hypermobility and temporomandibular disorders: inherited connective tissue disease as a model with maximum expression. J Orofac Pain 19:47-57.

de Kort LM, Verhulst JA, Engelbert RH, Uiterwaal CS, de Jong TP (2003). Lower urinary tract dysfunction in children with generalized hypermobility of joints. J Urol 170:1971-1974.

De Vos M, Nuytinck L, Verellen C, De Paepe A (1999). Preterm premature rupture of membranes in a patient with the hypermobility type of the Ehlers-Danlos syndrome. A case report. Fetal Diagn Ther 14:244-247.

Di Palma F, Cronin AH (2005). Ehlers-Danlos syndrome: correlation with headache disorders in a young woman. J Headache Pain 6:474-475.

Dolan AL, Mishra MB, Chambers JB, Grahame R (1997). Clinical and echocardiographic survey of the Ehlers-Danlos syndrome. Br J Rheum 36:459-462.

Dolan AL, Arden NK, Grahame R, Spector TD (1998). Assessment of bone in Ehlers Danlos syndrome by ultrasound and densitometry. Ann Rheum Dis 57:630-633.

134

Eisenbeiss C, Martinez A, Hagedorn-Greiwe M, Reinhardt DP, B‰otge B, Brinckmann J (2003). Reduced skin thickness: a new minor diagnostic criterion for the classical and hypermobility types of Ehlers-Danlos syndrome. Br J Dermatol 149:850-852.

El-Garf A, Mahmoud GA, Mahgoub EH (1998). Hypermobility among Egyptian children: prevalence and features. J Rheumatol 25:1003-1005.

el-Shahaly HA, el-Sherif AK (1991). Is the benign joint hypermobility syndrome benign? Clin Rheumatol 10:302-307.

Engelbert RHH, Uiterwaal CSPM, van de Putte E, Helders PJM, Sakkers RJB, van Tintelen P, Bank RA (2003). Pediatric generalized joint hypomobility and musculoskeletal complaints: a new entity? Clinical, biochemical, and osseal characteristics. Pediatrics 113:714-719.

Engelbert RHH, Kooijmans FTC, van Riet AMH, Feitsma TM, Uiterwaal CSPM, Helders PJM (2005). The relationship between generalized joint hypermobility and motor development. Pediatr Phys Ther 17:258-263.

Enomoto M, Li L, Aritake S, Nagase Y, Kaji T, Tagaya H, Matsuura M, Kaneita Y, Ohida T, Uchiyama M (2006). Restless legs syndrome and its correlation with other sleep problems in the general adult population of Japan. Sleep Biol Rhythms 4:153-159.

Everman DB, Robin NH (1998). Hypermobility syndrome. Pediatr Rev 19:111-117.

Fossey M, Libman E, Bailes S, Baltzan M, Schondorf R, Amsel R, Fichten CS (2004). Sleep quality and psychological adjustment in chronic fatigue syndrome. J Behav Med 27:581-605.

Gannon LM, Bird HA (1999). The quantification of joint laxity in dancers and gymnasts. J Sports Sci 17:743-750.

Gazit Y, Nahir AM, Grahame R, Jacob G (2003). Dysautonomia in the hypermobility syndrome. Am J Med 115:33-40.

Gedalia A, Press J, Klein M, Buskila D (1993). Joint hypermobility and fibromyalgia in schoolchildren. Ann Rheumat Dis 52:494-496.

Girotto JA, Malaisrie SC, Bulkely G, Manson PN (2000). Recurrent ventral herniation in Ehlers-Danlos syndrome. Plast Reconstr Surg 106:1520-1526.

Giunta C, Superti-Furga A, Spranger S, Cole WG, Steinmann B (1999). Ehlers-Danlos syndrome type VII: clinical features and molecular defects. J Bone Joint Surg 81:225-238.

Goldberg MJ (1987). "The Dysmorphic Child: An Orthopedic Perspective." Raven Press, New York; pp 247-263.

Golfier F, Peyrol S, Attia-Sobol J, Marret H, Raudrant D, Plauchu H (2001). Hypermobility type of Ehlers-Danlos syndrome: influence of pregnancies. Clin Genet 60:240-241.

Grahame R, Edwards JC, Pitcher D, Gabell A, Harvey W (1981). A clinical and echocardiographic study of patients with the hypermobility syndrome. Ann Rheum Dis 40:541-546.

Grahame R (1989). How often, when and how dose joint hypermobility lead to osteoarthritis? Br J Rheumatol 28:320.

Grahame R, Bird HA, Child A (2000). The revised (Brighton 1998) criteria for the diagnosis of benign joint hypermobility syndrome (BJHS). J Rheumatol 27:1777-1779.

Grahame R, Bird H (2001). British consultant rheumatologists' perceptions about the hypermobility syndrome: a national survey. Rheumatol 40:559-562.

Grahame R, Hakim AJ (2008). Hypermobility. Curr Opin Rheumatol 20:106-110.

Gulbahar S, Sahin E, Baydar M, Bircan C, Kizil R, Manisali M, Akalin E, Peker O (2006). Hypermobility syndrome increases the risk for low bone mass. Clin Rheumatol 25:511-514.

Gulsun M, Yilmaz MB, Pinar M, Tonbul M, Celik C, Ozdemir B, Dumlu K, Erbas M (2007). Thorax deformity, joint hypermobility and anxiety disorders. Saudi Med J 28:1840-1844.

Gurley-Green S (2001). Living with the hypermobility syndrome. Rheumatol 40:487-489.

Hagberg C, Berglund B, Korpe L, Andersson-Norinder J (2004). Ehlers-Danlos Syndrome (EDS) focusing on oral symptoms: a questionnaire study. Orthod Craniofac Res 7:178-185.

Hakim A, Grahame R (2003). Joint hypermobility. Best Pract Res Clin Rheumatol 17:989-1004.

Hakim AJ, Grahame R (2004). Non-musculoskeletal symptoms in joint hypermobility syndrome. Indirect evidence for autonomic dysfunction? Rheumatol 43:1194-1195.

Hakim AJ, Grahame R, Norris P, Hopper C (2005). Local anaesthetic failure in joint hypermobility syndrome. J R Soc Med 98:84-85.

Hall MG, Ferrell WR, Sturrock RD, Hamblen DL, Baxendale RH (1995). The effect of the hypermobility syndrome on knee joint proprioception. Br J Rheumatol 34:121-125.

Hampton T (2008). Improvements needed in management of temporomandibular joint disorders. JAMA 299:1119-1121.

Handler CE, Child A, Light ND, Dorrance DE (1985). Mitral valve prolapse, aortic compliance, and skin collagen in joint hypermobility syndrome. Br Heart J 54:501-508.

Hanioka T, Tanaka M, Ojima M, Shizukuishi S, Folkers K (1994). Effect of topical application of coenzyme Q10 on adult periodontitis. Mol Aspects Med 15:241-248.

Hasenbring M, Marienfeld G, Kuhlendahl D, Soyka D (1994). Risk factors of chronicity in lumbar disc patients. A prospective investigation of biologic, psychological, and social predictors of therapy outcome. Spine 19:2759-2765.

Hermanns-Lí T, PiÈrard G, Quatresooz P (2005). Ehlers-Danlos-like dermal abnormalities in women with recurrent preterm premature rupture of fetal membranes. Am J Dermatopathol 27:407-410.

Hordnes K (1994). Ehlers-Danlos syndrome and delivery. Acta Obstet Gynecol Scand 73:671-673.

Howes RG, Isdale IC (1971). The loose back: an unrecognized syndrome. Rheum Phys Med 11:72-77.

Hudson N, Starr MR, Esdaile JM, Fitzcharles MA (1995). Diagnostic associations with hypermobility in rheumatology patients. Br J Rheumatol 34:1157-1161.

Hunt RH, Choquette D, Craig BN, De Angelis C, Habal F, Fulthorpe G, Stewart JI, Turpie AGG, Davis P (2007). Approach to managing musculoskeletal pain: acetaminophen, cyclooxygenase-2 inhibitors, or traditional NSAIDs? Can Fam Phys 53:1177-1184.

Hyams JS (2004). Irritable bowel syndrome, functional dyspepsia, and functional abdominal pain syndrome. Adolesc Med Clinic 14:1-15.

Ignoto A, Ambrogio M, Distefano N, Presti C, Puglisi F, Vaccarella A, Nucifora R (2006). Acute para-esophageal hernia in Ehlers-Danlos Syndrome. Chir Ital 58:797-801.

Iosif CS, Bekassy Z, Rydhstrom H (1988). Prevalence of urinary incontinence in middle-aged women. Int J Gynaecol Obstet 26:255-259.

Jacome DE (1999). Headache in Ehlers-Danlos syndrome. Cephalalgia 19:791-796.

Jerosch J, Castro WH (1990). Shoulder instability in Ehlers-Danlos syndrome. An indication or surgical treatment? Acta Orthoped Belg 56:451-453.

Jonsson H, Valtysdottir ST (1995). Hypermobility features in patients with hand osteoarthritis. Osteoarthritis Cartilage 3:1-5.

Karaaslan Y, Haznedarogiu S, Ozturk M (2000). Joint hypermobility and primary fibromyalgia: a clinical enigma. J Rheum 27:1774-1776.

137

Karan A, Isikoglu M, Aksac B, Attar E, Eskiyurt N, Yalcin O (2004). Hypermobility syndrome in 105 women with pure urinary stress incontinence and in 105 controls. Arch Gynecol Obstet 269:89-90.

Keer R, Grahame R (2003). Hypermobility Syndrome: Recognition and Management for Physiotherapists. London, Butterworth Heinemann.

Khocht A, Calem B, Deasy M (2004). Use of anti-inflammatory medications in managing atypical gingivitis associated with hypermobile Ehlers-Danlos syndrome: a case report. J Periodontol 75:1547-1552.

Kiiholma P, Gronroos M, Nanto V, Paul R (1984). Pregnancy and delivery in Ehlers-Danlos syndrome. Role of copper and zinc. Acta Obstet Gynecol Scand 63: 437-439.

Kirk JA, Ansell BM, Bywaters EGL (1967). The hypermobility syndrome. Ann Rheum Dis 26:419-425.

Kobayasi T (2006). Dermal elastic fibres in the inherited hypermobile disorders. J Dermatol Sci 41:175-185.

Konvicka JJ, Meyer TA, McDavid AJ, Roberson CR (2008). Complementary/alternative medicine use among chronic pain clinic patients. J Perianesth Nurs 23:17-23.

Kosinski M, Janagap C, Gajria K, Schein J, Freedman J (2007). Pain relief and pain-related sleep disturbance with extended-release tramadol in patients with osteoarthritis. Curr Med Res Opin 23:1615-1626.

Kundermann B, Krieg JC, Schreiber W, Lautenbacher S (2004). The effect of sleep deprivation on pain. Pain Res Manag 9:25-32.

Lacy BE, Cash BD (2008). A 32-year-old woman with chronic abdominal pain. JAMA 299:555-565.

Larsson LG, Mudholkar GS, Braum J, Srivastava DK (1995). Benefits and liabilities of hypermobility in the back pain disorders of industrial workers. J Intern Med 238:461-467.

Leeuw M, Goossens ME, Linton SJ, Crombez G, Boersma K, Vlaeyen JW (2007). The fear-avoidance model of musculoskeletal pain: current state of scientific evidence. J Behav Med 30:77-94.

LÈtourneau Y, PÈrusse R, Buithieu H (2001). Oral manifestations of Ehlers-Danlos syndrome. J Can Dent Assoc 67:330-334.

Levy HP, Mayoral W, Collier K, Tio TL, Francomano CA (1999). Gastroesophageal reflux and irritable bowel syndrome in classical and hypermobile Ehlers-Danlos syndrome (EDS). Am J Hum Genet 65:A69.

Levy HP (2007). Ehlers-Danlos syndrome, hypermobility type. In: *GeneReviews*, http:// www.genetests.org/, last accessed 3/18/08.

Lewkonia RM (1986). Does generalised articular hypermobility predispose to generalised osteoarthritis? Clin Exp Rheumatol 4:115-119.

Lichtenstein IL, Shulman AG, Amid PK, Monttlor MM (1989). The tension-free hernioplasty. Am J Surgery 157:188-193.

Lichtenstein IL, Shulman AG, Amid PK (1991). Twenty questions about hernioplasty Am Surg 57:730-733.

Lind J, Wallenburg HCS (2002). Pregnancy and the Ehlers-Danlos syndrome: a retrospective study in a Dutch population. Acta Obstet Gynecol Scand 81:293-300.

Logan NS, Davies LN, Mallen EA, Gilmartin B (2005). Ametropia and ocular biometry in a UK university student population. Optom Vis Sci. 82:261-266.

Lugaresi E, Coccagna G, Tassinari CA, Ambrosetto C (1965). Polygraphic data on motor phenomena in the restless legs syndrome. Rivista di Neurologia 35:550-561.

Lumley MA, Jordan M, Rubenstein R, Tsipouras P, Evans MI (1994). Psychosocial functioning in the Ehlers-Danlos syndrome. Am J Med Genet 53:149-152.

Malfait F, Croucke P, Symoens S, Loeys B, Nuytinck L, De Paepe A (2005). The molecular basis of classic Ehlers-Danlos syndrome: a comprehensive study of biochemical and molecular findings in 48 unrelated patients. Hum Mutat 25:28-37.

Malleson PN, Connell H, Bennett SM, Eccleston C (2001). Chronic musculoskeletal and other idiopathic pain syndromes. Arch Dis Child 84:189-192.

Mallik AK, Ferrell WR, McDonald AG, Sturrock RD (1994). Impaired proprioceptive acuity at the proximal interphalangeal joint in patients with the hypermobility syndrome. Br J Rheumatol 33:631-637.

Mandell K, Griswold B, Francomano C, McDonnell N (2006). Sleep disturbance in Ehlers-Danlos syndromes: related to chronic pain or an independent entity. In: 56th Annual Meeting of the American Society of Human Genetics.

Mantle D, Wilkins RM, Preedy V (2005). A novel therapeutic strategy for Ehlers-Danlos syndrome based on nutritional supplements. Med Hypotheses 64:279-283.

Marnach ML, Ramin KD, Ramsey PS, Song SW, Stensland JJ, An KN (2003). Characterization of the relationship between joint laxity and maternal hormones in pregnancy. Obstet Gyn101:331-335.

Martin-Santos R, Bulbena A, Porta M, Gago J, Molina L, Duru, JC (1998). Association between joint hypermobility syndrome and panic disorder. Am J Psychiatry 155:1578-1583.

McDermott ML, Holladay J, Liu D, Puklin JE, Shin DH, Cowden JW (1998). Corneal topography in Ehlers-Danlos syndrome. J Cataract Refract Surg 24:1212-1215.

McDonnell NB, Gorman BL, Mandel KW, Schurman SH, Assanah-Carroll A, Mayer SA, Najjar SS, Francomano CA (2006). Echocardiographic findings in classical and hypermobile Ehlers-Danlos syndromes. Am J Med Genet A 140:129-136.

McIntosh LJ, Mallett VT, Frahm JD, Richardson DA, Evans MI (1995). Gynecologic disorders in women with Ehlers-Danlos syndrome. J Soc Gynecol Invest 2:559-564.

Meeus M, Nijs J, Meirleir KD (2007). Chronic musculoskeletal pain in patients with the chronic fatigue syndrome: a systematic review. Eur J Pain 11:377-386.

Milhorat TH, Bolognese PA, Nishikawa M, McDonnell NB, Francomano CA (2007). Syndrome of occipitoatlantoaxial hypermobility, cranial settling, and Chiari malformation type I in patients with hereditary disorders of connective tissue. J Neurosurg Spine 7:601-609.

Miller VJ, Zelster R, Yoeli Z, Bodner L (1997). Ehlers-Danlos syndrome, fibromyalgia and temporomandibular disorder: report of an unusual combination. Cranio 15:267-269.

Morales-Rosello J, Hernandez-Yago J, Pope M (1997). Type III Ehlers-Danlos syndrome and pregnancy. Arch Gynecol Obstet 261:39-43.

Morgan AW, Person SB, Davies S, Gooi HC, Bird HA (2007). Asthma and airways collapse in two heritable disorders of connective tissue. Ann Rheum Dis 66:1369-1373.

Murray KJ (2006). Hypermobility disorders in children and adolescents. Best Pract Res Clin Rheumatol 20:329-351.

Nematbakhsh A, Crawford AH (2004). Non-adjacent spondylolisthesis in Ehlers-Danlos syndrome. J Pediatr Orthop B 13:336-339.

Nijs J, Van Essche E, De Munck M, Dequeker J (2000). Ultrasonographic, axial, and peripheral measurements in female patients with benign hypermobility syndrome. Calcif Tissue Int 67:37-40.

Nijs J, Aerts A, De Meirleir K (2006). Generalized joint hypermobility is more common in chronic fatigue syndrome than in healthy control subjects. J Manipulative Physiol Ther 29:32-39.

Norton LA, Assael LA (1997). Orthodontic and temporomandibular joint considerations in treatment of patients with Ehlers-Danlos syndrome. Am J Othod Dentofac Orthop 111:75-84.

Norton PA, Baker JE, Sharp HC, Warenski JC (1995). Genitourinary prolapse and joint hypermobility in women. Obstet Gynecol 85:225-228.

140

Nualart Grollmus ZC, Morales Chavez MC, Silvestre Donat FJ (2007). Periodontal disease associated to systemic genetic disorders. Med Oral Patol Oral Cir Bucal 12:E211-E215.

Ofluoglu D, Gunduz OH, Kul-Panza E, Guven Z (2006). Hypermobility in women with fibromylagia syndrome. Clin Rheumatol 25:291-293.

O'Loughlin PF, Hodgkins CW, Kennedy JG (2008). Ankle sprains and instability in dancers. Clin Sports Med 27:247-262.

Osorio CD, Gallinaro AL, Lorenzi-Filho G, Lage LV (2006). Sleep quality in patients with fibromyalgia using the Pittsburgh Sleep Quality Index. J Rheumatol 33:1863-1865.

Parapia LA, Jackson C (2008). Ehlers-Danlos syndrome- a historical review. Br J Haematol 141:32-35.

Park DH, Ramakrishnan P, Cho TH, Lorenz E, Ecjk JC, Humphreys SC, Lim TH (2007). Effect of lower two-level anterior cervical fusion on the superior adjacent level. J Neurosurg Spine 7:336-340.

Pemberton JW, Freeman HM, Schepens CL (1966). Familial retinal detachment and the Ehlers-Danlos syndrome. Arch Ophthalmol 76:817-824.

Perez LA, Al-Shammari KF, Giannobile WV, Wang HL (2002). Treatment of periodontal disease in a patient with Ehlers-Danlos syndrome. A case report and literature review. J Periodontol 73:564-570.

Pesudovs K (2004). Orbscan mapping in Ehlers-Danlos syndrome. J Cataract Refract Surg 30:1795-1798.

Pountain G (1992). Musculoskeletal pain in Omanis, and the relationship to joint hypermobility and body mass index. Br J Rheum 31:81-85.

Rabago D, Best TM, Beamsley M, Patterson J (2005). A systematic review of prolotherapy for chronic musculoskeletal pain. Clin J Sport Med 15:376-380.

Raffa RB, Clark-Vetri R, Tallarida RJ, Wertheimer AI (2003). Combination strategies for pain management. Expert Opin Pharmacother 4:1697-1708.

Rajagopalan M, Kurian G, John J (1998). Symptom relief with amitriptyline in the irritable bowel syndrome. J Gastroenterol Hepatol 13:738-741.

Ranjbaran Z, Keefer L, Stepanski E, Farhadi A, Keshavarzian A (2007). The relevance of sleep abnormalities to chronic inflammatory conditions. Inflamm Res 56:51-57.

Reichert S, Riemann D, Plaschka B, Machulla HK (1999). Early-onset periodontitis in a patient with Ehlers-Danlos syndrome type III. Quintessence Int 30:785-790.

Rose GK (1990). Flat feet in children. BMJ 301:1330-1331.

Rose PS, Johnson CA, Hungerford DS, McFarland EG (2004). Total knee arthroplasty in Ehlers-Danlos syndrome. J Arthroplasty 19:190-196.

Rowe PC, Bou-Holaigah I, Kan JS, Calkins H (1995). Is neurally mediated hypotension an unrecognized cause of chronic fatigue? Lancet 345:623-624.

Rowe PC, Barron DF, Calkins H, Maumenee IH, Tong PY, Geraghty MT (1999). Orthostatic intolerance and chronic fatigue syndrome associated with Ehlers-Danlos syndrome. J Pediatr 135:494-499.

Russek LN (2000). Examination and treatment of a patient with hypermobility syndrome. Physical Therapy 4:386-398.

Sacheti A, Szemere J, Bernstein B, Tafas T, Schechter N, Tsipouras P (1997). Chronic pain is a manifestation of the Ehlers-Danlos syndrome. J Pain Symptom Manage 14:88-93.

Sakala EP, Harding MD (1991). Ehlers-Danlos syndrome type III and pregnancy. A case report. J Reprod Med 36:622-624.

Sapauskas B, Ambrozaitis KV, Tamasauskas A, Kontautas E (2007). Late radiographic findings after the anterior cervical fusion for the cervical subaxial compressive flexion and vertical compression injuries in young patients. Medicina (Kaunas) 43:542-547.

Sayar K, Arikan M, Yontem T (2002). Sleep quality in chronic pain patients. Can J Psychiatry 47:844-848.

Scott D, Bird H, Wright V (1979). Joint laxity leading to osteoarthritis. Rheumatol Rehabil 18:167-169.

Sevim S, Dagu O, Kaleagasi H, Aral M, Metin O, Camdeviren H (2004). Correlation of anxiety and depression symptoms in patients with restless legs syndrome: a population based survey. J Neurol Neurosurg Psychiatry 75:226-230.

Shariata A, Maceda JS, Hale DS (2008). High-fiber diet for treatment of constipation in women with pelvic floor disorders. Obstet Gynecol 111:908-913.

Shulman AG, Amid PK, Lichtenstein IL (1990). The "plug" repair of 1,402 recurrent inguinal hernia. Arch Surg 125.265-267.

Shulman AG, Amid PK, Lichtenstein IL (1992). Prosthetic mesh repair of femoral and recurrent inguinal hernias: the American experience. Ann R Coll Surg Engl 74:97-99.

Shulman AG, Amid PK, Lichtenstein IL (1992). The safety of mesh repair for primary inguinal hernias - results of 3,019 operations from five diverse surgical sources. Am Surg 58:255-257.

Siegel DM, Janeway D, Baum J (1998). Fibromyalgia syndrome in children and adolescents: clinical features at presentation and follow-up. Pediatrics 101:377-382.

Simmonds JV, Keer RJ (2008). Hypermobility and the hypermobility syndrome, part 2: assessment and management of hypermobility syndrome: illustrated via case studies. Manual Therapy 13:e1-e11.

Simpson MR (2006). Benign joint hypermobility syndrome: evaluation, diagnosis, and management. JAOA 106:531-536.

Slemenda C, Griswold BF, Sloper L, Francomano CA, McDonnell NB (2007). Postural orthostatic tachycardia is an age dependent manifestation of Ehlers-Danlos syndromes. In: 57th Annual Meeting of the American Society of Human Genetics.

Smith MS, Mitchell J, Corey L, Gold D, McCauley EA, Glover D, Tenover FC (1991). Chronic fatigue in adolescents. Pediatrics 88:195-202.

Solomon JA, Abrams L, Lichtenstein GR (1996). GI manifestations of EDS. Am J Gastroenterol 91:2282-2288.

Sorokin Y, Johnson MP, Rogowski N, Richardson DA, Evans MT (1994). Obstetric and gynecologic dysfunction in the Ehlers-Danlos syndrome. J Reprod Med 39:281-284.

Stanitski DF, Nadjarian R, Stanitski CL, Bawle E, Tsipouras P (2000). Orthopaedic manifestations of Ehlers-Danlos syndrome. Clin Ortho Rel Res 376:213-221.

Staud R (2007). Mechanisms of acupuncture analgesia: effective therapy for musculoskeletal pain? Curr Rheumatol Rep 9:473-481.

Steinmann B, Royce PM, Superti-Furga A (1993). The Ehlers-Danlos syndrome. In: *Connective Tissue and Its Heritable Disorders,* Royce PM, Steinmann B, eds. New York: Wiley-Liss, pp. 351-408.

Taylor DJ, Wilcox I, Russell JK (1981). Ehlers-Danlos syndrome during pregnancy: a case report and review of the literature. Obstet Gynecol Surv 36:277-281.

Unger ER, Nisenbaum R, Moldofsky H, Cesta A, Sammut C, Reyes M, Reeves WC (2004). Sleep assessment in a population-based study of chronic fatigue syndrome. BMC Neurol 4:6.

van de Putte EM, Uiterwaal CSPM, Bots ML, Kuis W, Kimpen JLLL, Engelbert RHH (2005). Is chronic fatigue syndrome a connective tissue disorder? A cross-sectional study in adolescents. Pediatrics 115:e415-e422.

van der Watt G, Laugharne J, Janca A (2008). Complementary and alternative medicine in the treatment of anxiety and depression. Curr Opin Psychiatry 21:37-42.

143

Verbraecken J, Declerck A, Van de Heyning P, De Backer W, Wouters EF (2001). Evaluation for sleep apnea in patients with Ehlers-Danlos syndrome and Marfan: a questionnaire study. Clin Genet 60:360-365.

Verhoeven JJ, Tuinman M, Van Dongen PW (1999). Joint hypermobility in African non-pregnant nulliparous women. Eur J Obstet Gynecol Reproduc Biol 82:69-72.

Volkov N, Nisenblat V, Ohel G, Gonen R (2007). Ehlers-Danlos syndrome: insights on obstetric aspects. Obstet Gynecol Surv 62:51-57.

Wang SM, Kain ZN, White PF (2008). Acupuncture analgesia: II. Clinical considerations. Anesth Analg 106:611-621.

Weinberg J, Doering C, McFarland EG (1999). Joint surgery in Ehlers-Danlos patients: results of a survey. Am J Orthop 28:406-409.

Wensor M, McCarty CA, Taylor HR (1999). Prevalence and risk factors of myopia in Victoria, Australia. Arch Ophthalmol 117:658-663.

Wenstrup RJ, Florer JB, Willing MC, Giunta C, Steinmann B, Young F, Susic M, Cole WG (2000). COL5A1 haploinsufficiency is a common molecular mechanism underlying the classical form of EDS. Am J Hum Genet 66:1766-1776.

Wenstrup RJ, Hoechstetter LB (2005). Ehlers-Danlos syndromes. In: "Management of Genetic Syndromes", 2nd ed., Cassidy SB, Allanson JE, eds. New York: Wiley-Liss, pp.211-223.

Westling L, Mattiasson A (1992). General joint hypermobility and temporomandibular joint derangement in adolescents. Ann Rheum Dis 51: 87-90.

Wynne-Davis R (1979). Familial joint laxity. Proc R Soc Med 64:689-690.

Yen JL, Lin SP, Chen MR, Niu DM (2006). Clinical features of Ehlers-Danlos syndrome. J Formos Med Assoc 105:475-480.

Zweers MC, Kucharekova M, Schalkwijk J (2005). Tenascin-X: a candidate gene for benign joint hypermobility syndrome and hypermobility type Ehlers-Danlos syndrome? Ann Rheum Dis 64:504-505.

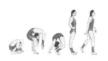

Notes

Notes

About The Author

Brad T. Tinkle, M.D., Ph.D., is a clinical and clinical molecular geneticist at Cincinnati Children's Hospital Medical Center (CCHMC).

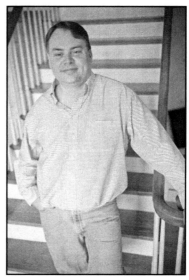

He specializes in caring for individuals with heritable connective tissue disorders such as Ehlers-Danlos syndromes, Marfan syndrome, osteogenesis imperfecta, and achondroplasia among the many. Dr. Tinkle serves as director of the Skeletal Dysplasia Center (CCHMC), co-director of the Marfan/Ehlers-Danlos syndrome clinic, as well as director of the Connective Tissue Clinic. Additionally, he serves as assistant director in the Clinical Molecular Genetics Laboratory at CCHMC.

Dr. Tinkle earned a bachelor's in science for engineering (BSE) in genetic engineering from Purdue University in 1989. He received his Ph.D. in Human Genetics from the George Washington University in the District of Columbia in 1995 and attended medical school at Indiana University and completed a pediatric/clinical genetics residency at CCHMC. He also finished a fellowship in clinical molecular genetics at CCHMC following residency.

Dr. Tinkle also currently serves on the Professional Advisory Network of the Ehlers-Danlos National Foundation.

Breinigsville, PA USA
16 August 2010
243683BV00002B/125/P